Understanding the Sick and the Healthy

Edited with an Introduction by N. N. Glatzer

HARVARD UNIVERSITY PRESS
CAMBRIDGE, MASSACHUSETTS
LONDON, ENGLAND

Franz Rosenzweig:

Understanding the Sick and the Healthy

A VIEW OF WORLD, MAN, AND GOD

With a New Introduction by Hilary Putnam

Introduction, 1999 copyright © 1999 by the President and Fellows of
Harvard College
English translation copyright 1954 by the Noonday Press, renewed
1982 by Farrar, Straus & Giroux, Inc.
German edition copyright © 1992 by Jüdischer Verlag im Suhrkamp
Verlag Frankfurt am Main
Printed in the United States of America

Published in German as *Das Büchlein vom gesunden und kranken
Menschenverstand* (1992)

First Harvard University Press paperback edition, 1999

Library of Congress Cataloging-in-Publication Data
Rosenzweig, Franz, 1886–1929.
    [Büchlein vom gesunden und kranken Menschenverstand.
English]
    Understanding the sick and the healthy : a view of world, man,
and God / Franz Rosenzweig : with a new introduction by
Hilary Putnam.
        p.   cm.
    Originally published: New York : Noonday Press, 1953.
    Includes bibliographical references.
ISBN 0-674-92119-4 (pbk.)
    1. Philosophy—Therapeutic use.   2. Life.   I. Title.
B3327.R63B8313   1999
181′.06—dc21   98-45818

My words are too difficult for you;
Therefore they appear to you as simple.
JUDAH HA-LEVI, *The Book of Kuzari*

Why is truth so woefully
Removed? To depths of secret banned?
None perceives in proper time! If we
But perceived in proper time, how bland
The truth would be, how fair to see!
How near and ready to our hand!
GOETHE, *Westöstlicher Diwan*

CONTENTS

1   *Introduction, 1999*

21   *Introduction*

35   *Preface to the "Expert"*

37   *Preface to the Reader*

39   Chapter One: THE ATTACK OF PARALYSIS

43   Chapter Two: VISIT AT THE SICKBED

47   Chapter Three: DIAGNOSIS

55   Chapter Four: THERAPY

59   Chapter Five: A PROFESSIONAL EXCHANGE OF
LETTERS

65   Chapter Six: THE CURE: FIRST WEEK

75   Chapter Seven: THE CURE: SECOND WEEK

85   Chapter Eight: THE CURE: THIRD WEEK

95   Chapter Nine: CONVALESCENCE

101   Chapter Ten: BACK TO WORK

105   *Epilogue to the "Expert"*

107   *Epilogue to the Reader*

109   *Notes*

115   *Acknowledgments*

117   *Chronology and Works*

Hilary Putnam

In terms of his depth, his originality, his immense learning, the power of his mind, and the compassion of his vision (not to mention his wide influence on non-Jewish as well as Jewish thinkers), Franz Rosenzweig ranks, along with Martin Buber and Emmanuel Levinas, as one of the most important Jewish thinkers of the twentieth century. Yet I must confess that it was not until I discovered this "little book" (literally translated, the original title is "The Little Book of Healthy and Sick Human Understanding") that I felt the power and the appeal of Rosenzweig's vision. In large part, this is because the book that made Rosenzweig famous, *The Star of Redemption,* is so *very* hard to read. The *Star* is an anti-Hegelian book written in what, at first blush, looks like Hegelian jargon—a critique of theology as conventionally understood, written in the form of what seems to be a theology, a critique of philosophy written in a prose which is not only learned but also highly idiosyncratic. Since this was the only work of Rosenzweig's that I had read, I did not expect to find him an author who could speak to my own condition. Yet this book (in addition to being an excellent preparation for reading the *Star*, that is, for understanding what the *Star* is really about, what it is "doing") presents the same vision in a radically different way. As a book intentionally written for non-philosophers, it eschews all philosophical jargon. Both the (anti-)philosophical vision and the religious vision are presented in a beautiful, simple, compelling prose. To my enormous surprise, I found *this* work reminding me of the last philosopher in the world I had expected to compare with Franz Rosenzweig, namely, Ludwig Wittgenstein, and I propose to explain a part of the illumination I find in Rosenzweig by presenting such a comparison.

Wittgenstein? Rosenzweig and *Wittgenstein?* Yet, on reflection, the comparison should not be as startling as it first seemed to me, for both thinkers are influenced by Kierkegaard[1] (if Wittgenstein was not a theist, he nonetheless had an obvious sympathy with religion), and both share a profoundly critical attitude toward the traditional philosophical search for a theory of the "essence" of things. I cannot imagine Wittgenstein reading through Rosenzweig's *The Star of Redemption*. Yet I can very easily imagine him reading and enjoying Rosenzweig's "little book" [*Büchlein*]. (It was Wittgenstein, after all, who remarked, "When Tolstoy just tells a story he impresses me infinitely more than when he addresses the reader",[2] and in the present book Rosenzweig adopts the manner of a storyteller.)

The roots of philosophical illusion

Although Wittgenstein says that the roots of philosophical illusion lie deep in our language and deep in us, he never attempts to provide a detailed account of those roots.[3] For Rosenzweig's purposes, however, it is essential to do just that. But why should Rosenzweig concern himself with philosophy at all? And especially why should he do this in a book which is explicitly written for non-philosophers, and which "experts", that is, philosophers, are explicitly warned away from reading?

One answer which does not work is that Rosenzweig is (only, or at least primarily) concerned with attacking *Hegelian* philosophy. Not only does this answer not fit the text (Rosenzweig mockingly describes ideas drawn from materialism, empiricism, positivism, Vaihinger's then well-known philosophy of "Als Ob" (As If), and not just Hegelian ideas), but it makes the paradox even more intractable. Could Rosenzweig really have supposed that the average German Jew of his time was in danger of becoming a convert to Hegelian metaphysics? But the answer is not really so hard to find. What philosophy represents here is not a technical subject at all, but a temptation to which all who think of themselves as religious may be subject at one time or another: the temptation to substitute *words*, especially words which have no religious content because they have no internal relation to a genuine religious life, for that kind of life. This is the very temptation that Kierkegaard was centrally concerned with combating. Kierkegaard didn't combat the temptation to substitute abstract talk for actually living the religious life because he imagined that most nineteenth-century Danish Christians were about to become metaphysicians—obviously not! Rosenzweig did not think that most twentieth-century German Jews were about to become Hegelians. These existentialist thinkers saw metaphysics as an exaggerated form of a disease to which we are all subject. It is this "disease" that the "physicians" in Rosenzweig's parable are out to diagnose and cure.

The absurdity of metaphysics

The similarity between Rosenzweig's criticism of philosophy and that of the later Wittgenstein extends also to their criticism of the metaphysician's search for an account of the "essence" of things as a search which is hopeless, not because it is too *difficult* to find the essence of things, but because the project is, in some sense, *absurd*. Both Wittgenstein and Rosenzweig direct us away from the chimera of a philosophical account of the "essence" of this or that to the ordinary use we make of our words. At the same time there is an obvious difference in their projects: for Wittgenstein, returning to the ordinary use of our words is to be aided by a precise and careful account of that use, by a "grammatical investigation". There is no such project in Rosenzweig; indeed, the present book, taken by itself, can seem—*must* perhaps seem, if taken apart from what Rosenzweig has written elsewhere—to be advising us to turn our backs on philosophy once and for all. Yet, as Wittgenstein recognized, if there is a way past philosophy in the sense of absurd metaphysics it must lead through philosophy in a different sense. Did Rosenzweig really not know this?

It is clear from what Rosenzweig wrote elsewhere (I shall give some examples later in this introduction) that he was fully aware of the need for another sort of philosophy. And I suspect, although I cannot of course prove, that the reason he decided not to publish the *Büchlein* may well have been precisely that, taken by itself, it seems excessively "anti-philosophical". Yet if one sees it as a Kierkegaardian work, one can understand both the quasi-fictional device it employs (narrating the course of a "disease" and its "cure" by a "sanatorium") and its deliberate one-sidedness.

The absurdity of metaphysics is, accordingly, not something that Rosenzweig *argues* for, as Wittgenstein *argues* that one or another metaphysical explanation of how it is possible to follow a rule, or possible to refer to things, or possible to do mathematics, collapses into absurdity when carefully probed, but rather something that he tries to make us *feel* by ironic redescription. (Although the Jewish religious sensibility is very different from the Christian, the devices of irony and parable remind one of *A Pilgrim's Progress*. Indeed, a possible alternative title for our "little book" might have been *A Patient's Progress*.) Thus Rosenzweig's first example of a philosopher's search for essences is the deliberately absurd one of a philosopher's seeking to know the essence of *a particular piece of butter.*

> Let us return to the example of the pound of butter. If we imagine the mental process of the buyer, we discover two possibilities: either he left home with the intention of buying, or he decided to do so when he passed the shop. Both possibilities have one thing in common—the slab of butter he finally buys is a very definite slab. Now, when did it become that particular piece? The instant the man at the counter sliced it. Or, perhaps, even earlier. If the latter, it may have happened when he discovered the butter in the shop window. What had it been previous to this? Nothing. And if the buyer did set out from home with the intention of buying butter, was it only butter in general that he had in mind? Certainly not. (p. 47)

4

Rosenzweig is well aware that philosophy journals do not contain papers about "the essence of butter". Yet one can easily imagine a present-day philosophy conference at which the following arguments are advanced:

> *Prof. A:* Suppose I want a slab of butter. It could be that, unknown to me, there is no butter in existence—it was all destroyed a few minutes ago. But I still want a slab of butter. That is true whether there actually exist slabs of butter or not. So the expression "a slab of butter" cannot have its normal function of referring to slabs of (actual) butter in "I want a slab of butter". What "I want a slab of butter" actually means is that I want there to be an X such that X is in my possession and X has the *attribute* Being a Slab of Butter. The expression "slab of butter" has what Frege called an "oblique" sense and reference. It really refers to the *attribute* Being a Slab of Butter when it occurs as the object of the verb "to want".

> *Prof. B:* Talk of "attributes" invokes immaterial, mysterious, hard-to-identify Abstract Entities. All that is mystery-mongering. What the sentence means might be expressed by saying, "I want-true the sentence 'I have a slab of butter'".

> *Prof. C:* What of third-person sentences, such as "John wants a slab of butter"?

> *Prof. B:* That means: John wants-true "I have a slab of butter" spoken by John.

> *Prof. C:* So "Pierre wants a slab of butter" means "Pierre wants-true the *English sentence* 'I have a slab of butter' spoken by Pierre"? What if Pierre doesn't know English?

> [Recall Rosenzweig: "If a philosopher, however, should turn his back on our slab of butter, claiming it cannot be butter, because the French call it *beurre*, the proper place for him would be an institution accommodating philosophers exclusively" (p. 53).]

> *Prof. D:* I suggest: "X wants a slab of butter" means "X wants-true some sentence which stands in the relation of synonymy to the following English sentence: 'I have a slab of butter'".

Of course, the participants at such a conference would probably deny that they are seeking the "essence" of butter. They would say that what they are looking for is "the right semantics for 'want-sentences'". But the notion of "the right semantics" in play here is quite obviously an *essentialist* one. The "right semantics" does not have to represent a way any actual speaker really *understands* such a sentence; it only has to correspond to a philosopher's "intuitions". Contemporary "semantics" is just old-fashioned metaphysics in disguise.

(It is instructive to compare the above Rube Goldberg accounts of the "semantics" of the verb "want" with Wittgenstein's straightforward remarks about wishes in *Philosophical Investigation,* §§440-441):

> §440: Saying "I should like an apple" does not mean: I believe an apple will quell my feeling of nonsatisfaction. *This* proposition is not an expression of a wish but of nonsatisfaction.

> §441: By nature and by a particular training, a particular education, we are disposed to give spontaneous expression to wishes in certain circumstances . . . In this game the question whether I know what I wish before my wish is fulfilled cannot arise at all. And the fact that some event stops my wishing does not mean that it fulfills it. Perhaps I should not have been satisfied if my wish had been satisfied.

What makes the butter I buy "the butter I wanted", if it is, is that I *describe* the butter I buy as "what I wanted". There is nothing in the butter itself, nor in the feelings of satisfaction/nonsatisfaction, and so on, which accompany the purchasing and eating of the butter, that makes the butter "the object of the desire" apart from what Wittgenstein calls "the language game" and Rosenzweig calls "the name". And "the name" functions perfectly well without the help of any essence. As Rosenzweig puts it:

> I transform the representation of my wish, as yet resembling the image in my memory, into what I see in the shop window. If we consider the matter without prejudice, we observe that after this change has taken place, nothing but the word "butter" remains the same. Is this all, then, nothing but a mere word, a name? All else has changed; the name remains. This is the first fact that must be stated. And what do we gain by such a statement? Above all, we make sure that no one is tempted to assume that the name is the "essence" of the thing. (p. 48)

6

But not nominalism

It is important not to take Rosenzweig's (or, again, Wittgenstein's) rejection of the search for essences as itself a positive metaphysical claim. The danger is, perhaps, more easily seen if we change our example of a metaphysical problem to, say, the famous "problem of personal identity"; indeed, Rosenzweig does clearly have this problem in mind when he writes, concerning "the courtship which precedes marriage",

> Since time must elapse, the answer is unavoidably given by another person than the one who was asked, and it is given to one who has changed since he asked it . . . a whole lifetime is involved in question and answer. The lovers dare not deny, not even Romeo and Juliet, that changes, involving both of them, will inevitably take place. Nevertheless they do not hesitate. Indeed, the man who proposes and the woman who replies do not reflect upon these vicissitudes. They cling to the unchangeable. What is the unchangeable? Unbiased reflection reveals once more that it is only a name. (p. 49)

If we make the mistake of supposing that Rosenzweig is here making a metaphysical claim, say, the metaphysical claim that there is nothing that the different things gathered under a name really have in common ("Nominalism"), this could be taken to say that what we refer to as a "person", as "John", say, or "Sally", is really a succession of different persons; indeed, the contemporary philosopher Derek Parfit has argued for just this point of view. According to Parfit,[4] each of my momentary selves, my "time-slices", has the right to be considered a different individual, and the idea that the self that will be called "Hilary Putnam" in a week's time is in any sense more "identical" to me than is a perfect stranger thousands of miles away is just a persistent illusion. But this view is just as metaphysical as the view it opposes, the view that there is some self-identical entity, some "substance", in traditional metaphysical terminology which is present as long as I am myself, and which is my "essence". In traditional religious thought, and also in the psychology of Descartes and other Rationalist philosophers, this substance was identified with an immaterial soul; but even if there are/were immaterial souls, could *they* not consist of different (immaterial) substances at different times? And would it make any difference to our personal identities if they did? And if there are no immaterial souls, does it make any difference to our personal identities if our bodies consist of different matter at different times?

Both Locke and Kant answered "no", but they did not deny, as Parfit does, that it makes sense to think of myself as the same person at different times. Nor does Rosenzweig. Indeed, as Rosenzweig points out, thinking this way is essential to our lives. As he writes, "common sense in action is concerned that the name, not the 'essence', remain" (p. 49). Or as Wittgenstein might have put it, "In this game the question whether the person we call 'Sally' is 'numerically identical' to her former self cannot arise at all".

I mentioned Locke and Kant, and if I may be permitted to digress, it is interesting to see how they each made a similar point. For Locke what makes me the very person who lived in such-and-such a town as a small boy, who went to such-and-such a high school and college and had such-and-such friends, who got married, worked at various places, wrote and said various things, etc., who did such-and-such and is now ashamed of it or proud of it, etc., is that I acknowledge those events as happening to me and my memories of them as my own. This is another way of making the point that "common sense in action" has no choice but to rely on the language game. For Kant, rational thought itself depends on the fact that I regard my thoughts, experiences, memories, etc., as all *mine* (that is, the fact that I prefix the "I think" to all of them, not just at the time but also retrospectively). To illustrate Kant's point, imagine yourself going through a very simple form of reasoning, say, "Boiling water hurts if you stick your finger in it; this is boiling water, so it will hurt if I stick my finger in this". If the "time-slice" of me that thought[5] "Boiling water hurts if you stick your finger in it" was one person, person A, and the "time-slice" that thought the minor premise "This is boiling water" is a different person, person B, and the person that thought the "conclusion", "It will hurt if I stick my finger in this", was yet a third person, person C, then that conclusion was not warranted—indeed, the sequence of thoughts was not an argument at all, since the thoughts were thoughts of different thinkers, none of whom had any reason to be

8

bound by what the others thought or had thought. We are *responsible* for what we have thought and done in the past, responsible *now*, intellectually and practically, and that is what makes us *thinkers*, rational agents in a world, at all. Kant, like Locke, can be seen as making the point that the "game" of thinking of my thoughts and actions at different times as *mine* does not depend on a metaphysical premise about "self-identical substances", and is nonetheless a game that we cannot opt out of as long as we are engaged in "common sense in action". Whereas Nominalism leaves us without any coherent conception of ourselves and our lives, *rejecting the question* that both the Rationalist Psychologist and the Nominalist try to answer directs our attention back to the conceptions that really inform those lives. These thinkers insist that the question, "How many self-identical substances do I consist of" is a question that diverts our attention away from the real issue, the issue of what is required for "common sense in action" [*der gesunde Menschenverstand in seinem Handeln*].

God

Rosenzweig is a *religious* thinker. The question he is concerned with—concerned with *vitally*, as a living practical question—is, What does "common sense in action" mean for a religious human being? By treating Man, the World, and God as three "mountains" that his "patient" glimpses from his sanatorium, Rosenzweig means to suggest that a proper relation to God no more depends on a *theory*, on an intellectual conception of what God "really is", or a grasp of the "essence" of God, than a proper relation to other human beings or to the world depends on a theory of man or the world. Again, a comparison with Wittgenstein may help in grasping the thought. In his masterly exposition and development of Wittgenstein's thought, *The Claim of Reason*,[6] Stanley Cavell interprets Wittgenstein as finding a "truth in skepticism", albeit one whose significance the skeptic distorts and misunderstands. It is true that we do not "know" that there is a world and that there are other people, on Cavell's interpretation, but not because (this is the skeptic's misunderstanding) we "don't know" these things. In ordinary circumstances, circumstances in which neither doubt nor justification is called for, our relation to the familiar things in our environment, the pen in our hand or the person in pain whom we are consoling, is not one of either "knowing" or "not knowing". Rather, Cavell suggests, it is one of *acknowledging* (or, sadly, failing to acknowledge). Our task is not to acquire a "proof" that "there is an external world" or that our friend is in pain, but to *acknowledge* the world and our friend. I suggest that we read Rosenzweig, the religious thinker, as adding that it is our task to acknowledge God (indeed, as a profoundly religious thinker, albeit also a profoundly humanist thinker, he does not think one can acknowledge any one of the three—God, Man, and World—as they demand to be acknowledged unless one acknowledges the other two). But like Cavell's Wittgenstein, Rosenzweig insists that acknowledging is not a matter of knowledge.

Although he has a religious sensibility,[7] Wittgenstein never calls himself a "theist". But it is clear that for him, too, a religion, if it is to have any value, cannot be a *theory:*

> It strikes me that a religious belief could only be something like a passionate commitment to a system of reference. Hence, although it's *belief,* it's really a way of living, or a way of assessing life. It's passionately seizing hold of *this* interpretation. Instruction in a religious faith, therefore, would have to take the form of a portrayal, a description, of that system of reference, while at the same time being an appeal to conscience [*ein in's-Gewissen-reden*]. And this combination would have to result in the pupil himself, of his own accord, passionately taking hold of the system of reference. It would be as though someone were first to let me see the hopelessness of my situation and then show me the means of rescue until, of my own accord, or not at any rate led to it by my *instructor,* I ran to it and grasped it.[8]

Fear of life and fear of death

It is important that Rosenzweig's passionate attack on the quest for essences—whether the quest be for an essence of Man, an essence of the World, or a grasp of the very essence of God—is not an attack on *wonder.* As Rosenzweig writes, "Were it a question of this gift alone, this capacity to wonder, philosophy's rightful claim to superiority could not be disputed" (p. 39). But wonder, Rosenzweig points out, however extensively (and peculiarly) it may be cultivated by philosophy, is not originally a particularly philosophical activity. Thus, almost immediately after the passage I just quoted, Rosenzweig continues, "But be that as it may, how does our philosopher know of wonder? In any case, where does he obtain the word? Does not the non-philosophizing half of mankind also wonder? The wonder of a child? The wonder of a savage? Does not wonder overcome them a hundred times—even oftener than the philosopher?" (pp. 39–40).

In that extraordinary thing called "ordinary" life, wonder arises and dissolves in the flow of life itself. Even as lovers wonder at each other, "the solution and dissolution of their wonder is at hand—the love which has befallen them. They are no longer a wonder to each other; they are in the very heart of wonder". And life "becomes numb in the face of death—and dies. The wonder is unravelled. And it was life itself that brought the solution" (p. 40).

As Rosenzweig sees it, the philosopher is a being who is incapable of accepting the process of life and what he calls "the passing of the numbness wonder has brought". Such a relief comes too slowly. The philosopher

> does not permit his wonder, stored as it is, to be released into the flow of life. Of necessity, he must hook the "problem" from where he stands. He has forcibly extracted thought's "object" and "subject" from the flow of life and he entrenches himself within them. Wonder *stagnates* [emphasis added], is perpetuated in the motionless mirror of his meditation; that is in the subject. He has it well-hooked; it is securely fastened, and it persists in his benumbed immobility. The stream of life has been replaced by something submissive—statuesque, subjugated. (pp. 40–41)

A number of critics of the traditional metaphysical enterprise have noted that the philosopher seeks an imaginary position, one outside the flow of time. He seeks to view everything, even himself, as if he were an "outsider"; he seeks to view the world as if he were not *in* it, to view it "from sideways on", as John McDowell has put it.[9] By describing this imaginary position as a place outside the current, outside the demands of life and the flow of time, Rosenzweig suggests that this sort of philosophy stems from a "fear to live" (p. 102). But at the close of *Under-*

standing the Sick and the Healthy, just before the epilogues, Rosenzweig gives a deeper diagnosis:

> We have wrestled with the fear to live, with the desire to step outside the current; now we may discover that reason's illness was merely an attempt to elude death. Man, chilled in the full current of life, sees, like that famous Indian prince, death waiting for him. So he steps outside of life. If living means dying, he prefers not to live. (p. 102)

It is, of course, easy for a healthy young man to call for the courage to face life, and even to face death. But, as is well known, Rosenzweig displayed his ability to live up to the demands of his own existential philosophy in a most remarkable way. *Understanding the Sick and the Healthy* was finished in July 1921. Early in 1922 the first signs of Lou Gehrig's disease appeared, and by the end of the year he was already experiencing difficulty in speaking and writing. Within a few years, he was reduced to a condition resembling that of the physicist Stephen Hawking—virtually paralyzed and forced to communicate by means of eye-blinks. (His wife would recite the alphabet, and he would spell out words by blinking at the letter he wanted.) Yet, under *these* conditions, he remained the intellectual leader of the school for adult Jewish education that he founded, translated the Bible from Hebrew into German together with Martin Buber, and produced a flood of fascinating letters and papers—letters, one must say, which remain full of confidence and free of self-pity right to the end! One's appreciation of Rosenzweig's own life attitude can only be deepened by observing how he managed to realize that attitude, and to live life to the fullest, under such a terrible handicap.

The new thinking is "speaking thinking"

I claimed earlier that it is clear from what Rosenzweig wrote elsewhere that he is not simply "anti-philosophical". Rather, he is concerned with calling for a different sort of philosophy, an existential philosophy which he refers to as simply "the new thinking". (In an epilogue to *The Star of Redemption* he lists, in addition to himself, a number of contemporaries as exponents of the "new thinking", including Martin Buber, Ferdinand Eber, Hans Ehrenberg, and Victor von Weizsäcker.[10]) But the new thinking is not the subject of *Understanding the Sick and the Healthy*—not *explicitly*, that is. What this little book artfully depicts is a certain religious attitude, one characterized by a profound but undogmatic acknowledgement of man, world, and God. It would be contrary to Rosenzweig's whole spirit to explain what that means by offering a blueprint. But before saying a word about Rosenzweig's Judaism, I wish to say a word or two about the kind of philosophy that Rosenzweig recommends in place of the kind of philosophy he so brilliantly satirizes. In this section, then, my quotations will come not from the present work but from a wonderful selection of Rosenzweig's letters and writings that Nahum Glatzer assembled to "present" Franz Rosenzweig's life and thought.[11]

It is clear from those letters and writings that the "new thinking" is continuous with the trajectory of Rosenzweig's life. I am not only alluding to the courage and the sense of adventure Rosenzweig displayed under terrible adversity. Even before the onset of his paralyzing illness, in a letter to Friedrich Meinecke dated August 30, 1920, in which he rejects the offer of a university lectureship, Rosenzweig exemplifies the attitudes he had argued for in *The Star of Redemption,* as well as in *Understanding the Sick and the Healthy.*

> The one thing I wish to make clear is that scholarship no longer holds the center of my attention, and that my life has fallen under the rule of a "dark drive" which I'm aware that I merely *name* by calling it "my Judaism" . . . The man who wrote *The Star of Redemption* . . . is of a very different caliber from the author of *Hegel and the State.*[12] Yet when all is said and done, the new book is only—a book. I don't attach any undue importance to it. The small—at times exceedingly small—thing called [by Goethe] "demand of the day" which is made upon me in my position at Frankfurt, I mean . . . the struggles with people and conditions, have now become the core of my existence . . . Now I only inquire when I find myself *inquired of.* Inquired of, that is, by *men* rather than by scholars . . . [T]he questions asked by human beings have become increasingly important to me.

This distinction between the questions of scholars and the questions of men was central to Rosenzweig's "new thinking". In lieu of attempting an overview of the approach that Rosenzweig had in mind by that term, I shall list a few highlights:

(1) *The new thinking is "speaking thinking"*. As Rosenzweig explains this idea,

the difference between the old and the new, the "logical" and the "grammatical" thinking,[13] does not lie in the fact that one is silent while the other is audible, but the fact that the latter needs another person and takes time seriously—actually, these two things are identical. In the old philosophy, "thinking" means thinking for no one else and speaking to no one else (and here, if you prefer, you may substitute "everyone" or the well-known "all the world" for "no one"). But "speaking" means speaking to some one and thinking for some one. And this some one is always a quite definite some one, and he has not merely ears, like "all the world", but also a mouth.[14]

What Rosenzweig means by this is that, in the active engagement with the *lived* philosophical or theological problems of another human being that he calls "speaking thinking", a speaker does not know in advance what he will say—or if, indeed, he will say anything: "Speech is bound by time and nourished by time and it neither can nor wants to abandon this element. It does not know in advance just where it will end. It takes its cues from others. In fact, it lives by virtue of another's life, whether that other is the one who listens to a story, answers in the course of a dialogue, or joins in a chorus".[15] In the same place, Rosenzweig daringly criticizes both Plato's dialogues and the Gospels because in those writings "the thinker knows his thoughts in advance", and (in the Platonic dialogues) the other is only raising the objections the author thought of himself: "This is why the great majority of philosophical dialogues—including most of Plato's—are so tedious. In actual conversations something happens".

(2) *Theology as well as philosophy must be humanized*. According to Rosenzweig, "Theological problems must be translated into human terms, and human problems brought into the pale of theology".[16]

(3) *We need "readiness" rather than "plans"*. The task that Rosenzweig undertook to make his life work, his "vocation" in the most serious sense, was nothing less than to restore a meaningful Jewish life in a Western country, Weimar Germany, in which Jews were rapidly forgetting their Jewishness. He wanted this restoration to be undogmatic, and,

although his was a deeply *religious* vocation, he wanted to revive *all* forms of Jewish learning, secular as well as religious. This is a task which he saw as possessing "unlimited" importance, since, for a religious Jew, it is a part of the everlasting task of preserving a "bridge" between man and God (and the image of a "bridge" is one of Rosenzweig's favorite metaphors for revelation, which he construes as an ongoing process, something that happens in each religiously lived life). At the same time, it is a task for a particular historical moment. Remarking on both these aspects, Rosenzweig writes:[17]

> What is intended to be of limited scope can be carried out according to a limited, clearly outlined plan—it can be "organized". The unlimited cannot be attained by organization. That which is distant can be attained only through that which is nearest at the moment. Any "plan" is wrong to begin with—simply because it is a plan. The highest things cannot be planned; for them readiness is everything. Readiness is the one thing we can offer to the Jewish individual within us, the individual we aim at.

And he adds:

> Only the first gentle push of the will—and "will" is almost too strong a word—that first quite gentle push we give ourselves when in the confusion of the world we quietly say, "we Jews", and by that expression commit ourselves to the eternal pledge that, according to an old saying, makes every Jew responsible for every other Jew. Nothing more is assumed than the simple resolve to say once: "Nothing Jewish is alien to me"—and this is in itself hardly a resolve, scarcely anything more than a small impulse to look around oneself and into oneself. What each will then see no one can venture to predict.

The Judaism of *Understanding the Sick and the Healthy* and the Judaism of the *Star*

Although Rosenzweig's conception of the "new thinking" first found expression in his magnum opus, *The Star of Redemption,* the Judaism of *Understanding the Sick and the Healthy* is more appealing in certain respects than that of the *Star.* However, certain important characteristics are common to both. Neither work asks the reader to subscribe to particular dogmas or to a particular orthodoxy.

"The presentness of the miracle of revelation is and remains its *content;* its historicity, however, is its ground and warrant".[18] The first part of this sentence formulates a point of agreement with the dialogic philosophy of Rosenzweig's good friend Martin Buber; the second part insists that subjective experiences of presentness must show their meaning and warrant in history, which is something Buber never says.[19] Judaism must not be reduced to a dead set of observances, or even to a modern set of slogans or an ideology:

> It would be necessary [for the person who has succeeded in saying "nothing Jewish is alien to me"] to free himself from those stupid claims that would impose "Juda-ism" on him as a canon of definite, circumscribed "Jewish duties" (vulgar orthodoxy), or "Jewish tasks" (vulgar Zionism), or—God forbid—"Jewish ideas" (vulgar liberalism).[20]

On the other hand, Judaism is nothing without historic continuity. Whereas Buber constantly dichotomizes, separating Judaism and, in fact, every religion, into a meaningful element which is reduced to an a-conceptual and unconceptualizable moment of dialogic relationship, the famous I/Thou moment, and a meaningless shell of dogmas and legislations, Rosenzweig stresses interdependence. Legislation [*Gesetz*], Rosenzweig tells Buber in a famous open letter,[21] may not have religious meaning, but it always has the potential to become something more than *Gesetz,* to become *Gebot* [divine bidding]. After all, education, which Buber values as much as Rosenzweig, is not a matter of continuous rapturous "I/Thou" experiences. But we go through the "dry" spells, the preliminaries, the study of ancient languages, the acquisition of facts, and so on, for the sake of what they make possible: the genuine *learning* which justifies all the hard work that came before. Similarly, keeping a "mitzvah" (a part of the Jewish Law) *can*, as a result of our "inertia", seem mere legislation, mere *Gesetz,* but as a result of our study and devotion, our attentiveness and openness to the divine, it can also become a command, a *Gebot.* The holy is not to be set simply in *opposition* to the profane, the "I/Thou" moments in opposition to the "I/It" moments, legislation simply in opposition to commandment.

In the present work the idea that the holy is not simply in opposition to the profane is expressed as a denial that the Jewish holiday is to be thought of as in opposition to the work day. We see this in the chapter entitled "Convalescence" (Chap. 9), when Rosenzweig writes: "It is through the holiday that the work day receives its definition. We must bear in mind that we are not dealing with something entirely distinct from the weekday world as though the serious side of life were now replaced by the elation of art" (p. 96).

For Rosenzweig, the importance of the Jewish holidays, the feasts and the fasts, lies precisely in their ability to relate the one who observes them to life as a whole: "Insofar as the holiday is exceptional, it merely confirms the work day. There is no superior content to the holiday. The holiday does not seek that which is absent from the work day, does not know what the work day is not capable of recognizing. It does, however, state explicitly and as a whole those things which the latter expresses only partially and occasionally. God, man, and the world are the content of the holiday, and in a perfectly everyday manner" (p. 96).

The very next sentences express the attitude Rosenzweig advocates with great beauty:

> The holiday knows as little as the sane, healthy work day, what God, man and the world "are". The holiday does not permit their "essences" to be disputed. It knows no remote God, no isolated man, no fenced-in world. God, man, and the world are for it in constant motion; they are in transition, the three of them constantly joining and interweaving and separating. The undulations of beseeching and receiving, receiving and thanking, go on incessantly. Man asks, God gives, the world receives and thanks—and then man asks anew. There can be no dead season, no merely localized pulsation here; the process must be continual. The holiday cannot pretend to isolate any of the three elements. It must do without the spectacle of drama, because unfortunately drama remains mere spectacle.

In *The Star of Redemption*, however, there is another aspect, one which disappears in the present book and, indeed, in almost all of Rosenzweig's later writing.[22] This aspect is far more Hegelian than Rosenzweig acknowledges; it seems to me to be the remnant of his former Hegelianism. It is the idea that two and only two religions—Judaism and Christianity—have genuine significance. Indeed, one may say that he grants these two religions *metaphysical* significance.

The most unfortunate aspects of *The Star of Redemption* are, in fact, its polemical remarks about religions other than these two—its scorn for Islam, for Hinduism, and so on. What Rosenzweig does in the *Star* is retain the Hegelian idea of a "world historic" religion, arguing that Christianity is *the* world historic religion par excellence, the one fated to bring "pagan" mankind to theism, and invent a new and contrasting metaphysical dignity for Judaism—the dignity of being the only "ahistoric" religion, not ahistoric in the sense of never changing, but ahistoric in the sense that, in some metaphysical way, the changes are not "real" changes. In effect, it is as if there were an *essence* of Judaism which did not change, much as Rosenzweig would object to that formulation. In effect, the "world-historic" religion, Christianity, is a witness to the truth of the "ahistoric" Judaism.

Given that in his best moments Rosenzweig beautifully attacks both essentialism and historicism, I find this aspect of the *Star* depressing, and the fact that it is wholly absent in this little book (and virtually absent from his later writing) something to be thankful for.

Above all, Rosenzweig sought to nourish an undogmatic, pluralistic, Jewish revival. He sought to teach that we are always in the presence of God, that there is essentially just one commandment, the commandment to love God,[23] and only one thing to ask for in prayer, the strength to meet "the small—at times exceedingly small—thing called "demand of the day" with courage and confidence. His Preface to the Reader welcomes the reader as if he or she were an old schoolmate about to enter his house for a visit. The reader to whom this book speaks will never forget the visit.

NOTES

1 For a profound account of this influence, see James Conant's "Putting Two and Two Together: Kierkegaard, Wittgenstein and the Point of View for Their Work as Authors", in Timothy Tessin and Mario von der Ruhr, eds., *Philosophy and the Grammar of Religious Belief* (New York: St. Martin's Press, 1995).

2   Norman Malcolm, *Ludwig Wittgenstein: A Memoir* (London: St. Martin's Press, 1962), p. 43.

3   But see Stanley Cavell's *The Claim of Reason* (Oxford: Oxford University Press, 1979), especially Part IV, for such an account in a Wittgensteinian spirit.

4   Derek Parfit, *Reasons and Persons* (Oxford: Oxford University Press, 1987).

5   Of course, the idea of "time-slice" *thinking* is incoherent. Thought requires time as well as dispositions of various kinds. Therefore the idea that all my "time-slices" are *selves* has only the appearance of sense. And giving the time-slices "thickness"—say, thinking of them as one minute thick—won't help either. Ascribing dispositions to a "time-slice" lacks even the appearance of sense.

6   Cavell, *The Claim of Reason.*

7   Wittgenstein famously remarked in a conversation with Drury, "I am not a religious person, but I cannot help seeing every problem from a religious point of view"(!). From *Ludwig Wittgenstein: Personal Recollections,* ed. Rush Rhees (Oxford: Oxford University Press, 1991), p. 94.

8   Wittgenstein, *Culture and Value* (Chicago: University of Chicago Press, 1980), p. 64.

9   John McDowell, in "Non-Cognitivism and Rule-Following", reprinted in his *Mind, Value, and Reality* (Cambridge, Mass.: Harvard University Press, 1998). See p. 207.

10   See "The New Thinking" (pp. 190–208), in *Franz Rosenzweig: His Life and Thought,* presented by Nahum Glatzer (New York: Schocken Books, 1961), p. 200. This section is a translation by Glatzer of "Das Neue Denken", supplementary notes to *The Star of Redemption.* Rosenzweig, *Kleinere Schriften,* pp. 377–398 (Berlin: Schocken Verlag, 1937).

11   *Franz Rosenzweig: His Life and Thought.*

12   An earlier book of Rosenzweig's, a scholarly study of Hegel's political philosophy.

13   I find it astounding that Rosenzweig employs the very terminology that Wittgenstein introduces when he distinguishes between looking to "logic" to solve philosophical problems and conceiving of his investigation as a "grammatical" one (cf. *Philosophical Investigations,* esp. §108 and §122).

14 "The New Thinking", in *Franz Rosenzweig: His Life and Thought,* p. 200.

15 Ibid., p. 199.

16 Ibid., p. 201.

17 "On Being a Jewish Person", in *Franz Rosenzweig: His Life and Thought,* p. 222. This section, pp. 214–227 of the volume, is Glatzer's translation of a portion of *Bildung und keine Ende,* an open letter on education, *Kleinere Schriften,* pp. 79–93.

18 *The Star of Redemption,* p. 183.

19 The idea of seeing this formulation as expressing agreement and disagreement with Buber was suggested to me by Man Lung Cheng.

20 "On Being a Jewish Person", p. 222. "Liberalism" here refers to what is called "Reform Judaism" in the United States.

21 *On Jewish Learning* (New York: Schocken, 1955).

22 I mean to suggest not that Rosenzweig changed his mind on this aspect of his thinking, but simply that it ceased to preoccupy him.

23 "God's first word to the soul that unlocks itself to him is 'love me'". *Star,* p. 177. On page 176, Rosenzweig describes the commandment to love God as essentially the only commandment.

Franz Rosenzweig wrote this little book in July, 1921. His major work, *The Star* of *Redemption,* written while in military service at the Balkan front, had just been published. The two-volume work on Hegel's political doctrines *(Hegel and the State)* which had been issued several months previously had caused discussion among political scientists and modern historians.

Rosenzweig had not planned to build on these foundations a career as a scholarly writer. He felt that his writings had served their purpose in preparing the ground for extensive communal activities. "I see my future only in life, not any more in writing," he says in a letter to Martin Buber.[1]

The living, spoken word was to replace the written one. Professor Friedrich Meinecke, celebrated historian, had offered Rosenzweig a lectureship at the University of Berlin. In rejecting the offer, Rosenzweig confided to Meinecke that scholarship no longer appeared to him as an end in itself; it had become a service—and not a service to ideas and disciplines but to human beings. Scientific curiosity and the omniverous appetite for knowledge belonged to the past. He now wanted to confront human beings (and scholars only insofar as they were human beings), whose search for knowledge cannot be answered by experts working within well-defined disciplines, but by men who are ready to use their knowledge in the service of man.[2]

To the dismay of his academic friends and his bourgeois family, Rosenzweig chose the unconventional field of adult education—unconventional for a man who could have found something "higher"—and settled in Frankfort on the Main as the head of the *Freies Jüdisches Lehrhaus*. This free house of Jewish studies which provided an open forum for the discussion of Jewish, philosophical, sociological and simply human issues, was introduced by Rosenzweig with a pamphlet entitled *On Education* [*Bildung und kein Ende*]. The *Lehrhaus* was to become the scene of activities such as he describes in his letter to Professor Meinecke.

From January to March, 1921, Rosenzweig taught a course in philosophy at the *Lehrhaus*, in which he dealt with such problems as knowledge and belief, end and beginning, action and suffering, soul and body, life and death. In a seminar running concurrently, Rosenzweig discussed background material for these lectures, particularly the writings of German idealism from Kant to Hegel. These philosophers were treated polemically. In opposition to the advocates of pure thought and critical idealism, Rosenzweig expounded his "New Thinking." This he indicated in the subtitle to the course: "About the use of common sense" [*Vom Gebrauch des gesunden Menschenverstandes.*] The term "common sense" is much in evidence in *The Star of Redemption,* particularly in the polemics against German Idealism.

The Star of Redemption had now been in the hands of the reader and its author had good reason for thinking the public would find it difficult. Rosenzweig, therefore, welcomed the invitation of an enterprising publisher (Fromann) to present his philosophy in a more popular manner. He felt he should allow himself this much of a deviation from his new way of life. The book was to be called *Das Büchlein vom gesunden und kranken Menschenverstand* (The little book of common sense and sick reason). The *Lehrhaus* lectures and especially the seminar, where

Rosenzweig could test the comprehensibility of his views, served as a preparation for the writing of the *Büchlein*.

Rosenzweig's changed attitude to writing is reflected in the style of this treatise. This well-composed and at times solemn little book has careless prefaces and epilogues; in certain sections we encounter a rough boyishness (as in the treatment of the "as if" theory), occasional innuendoes against "philosophy" when only German Idealism is meant. The mode of address is in several places either unnecessarily aggressive, or unnecessarily pedagogical.

When the *Star* was completed, Rosenzweig thought of the remaining years of his life as a gift bestowed on him. He compared his state of mind, at thirty-two, with Goethe's feelings on his eighty-second birthday, when he had finally completed the manuscript of *Faust*. This additional time granted him should be accepted with reverence, filled with meaningful action: "each day's demand" should be realized as it presents itself. The publisher's invitation to present his philosophy did not coincide with his own inner necessity to speak. Every argument in favor of publication was outweighed by his fear of placing in the reader's hands a book written "on request." One month after the completion of the manuscript Rosenzweig sent a copy to a friend and wrote that he had not yet decided to publish it. A short time later he withdrew the manuscript, giving carbon copies to friends.[3]

The book is now published a generation after it was written, in another part of the world and in a tongue alien to the author's own.

The reasons for silence and withdrawal are no longer valid. Rosenzweig's name has grown in significance since his death in 1929. His works are discussed in many lands, in many languages, and by men of different faiths and philosophical convictions. His conduct during eight years of almost total paralysis made his life an example of personal heroism. Any additional record, therefore, of his understanding of men, world and God can no longer be overlooked.

The biographical position of the book is not unimportant. It was the last essay which Rosenzweig wrote as a healthy man. The adherent of the old, speculative, conceptual philosophic systems is treated as a paralytic patient being cured by the New Thinking. Two or three months after the book was completed Rosenzweig noticed in himself certain irregularities of muscular movement—symptoms of a paralysis which turned the young, vigorous man into an invalid deprived of movement and speech. We cannot know therefore whether the employment of the paralysis motif in the book is a mere coincidence or the ironic expression of a premonition on the author's part. Be that as it may, the book is the utterance of a man standing at life's crossroads. As such it is more than the original publisher intended it to be. And more, indeed, than the author himself could have consciously realized.

The English title of the book, *Understanding the Sick and the Healthy,* has been chosen as an indication of the importance which the author attached to his images. The dissolution of the world of experience in the process of consciousness (Idealism in general), the deduction of everything from thought and the ego (Fichte), the treatment of the thinking subject as something abstract (Kant), the disappearance of the "unhappy consciousness" in the dialectic of Reason (Hegel), are not viewed by Rosenzweig as mere philosophical errors but as a sickness of the whole man. Equally, the application of "common sense" is not meant to be a correction of the mind only but an expression of the health of man as a whole.

II

Rosenzweig's target in *Understanding the Sick and the Healthy* is German idealist philosophy which "reduces the world" to the perceiving "self." Such a philosophy, assuming that the world must be different from what it "appears" to be, inquires into the "essence" [*Wesen*] of things in order to establish what they are "actually" or "essentially" [*eigentlich*]. The New Thinking, grounded in common sense, traces experience of the world back to the world, experience of God back to God. As opposed to idealism, the New Thinking recognizes world, man and God—"the proper subjects of all philosophy"—as the three ultimate parts of reality.

Contrary to the teaching of idealism, our thoughts and ideas about things are not fundamental reality; the laws of thought are not identical with the laws of reality, as Kant maintained. The thinking subject is not an abstract being; mind and consciousness cannot be understood mathematically. Common sense regards individual human existence with utter seriousness. Here the "thinking individual" is personally involved both in the question and in the answer; his thinking does not concern his mind only but has an existential relevance.

The term "common sense" is usually associated with Thomas Reid (1710-1796) and his critique of Hume's epistemological radicalism and Berkeley's subjective idealism and immaterialism. In opposing Hume, Reid speaks of instinctive, intuitive, original principles and beliefs (such as the notion of an external world and the soul) which we know through experience; these principles of common sense, the bases of our knowledge, are older and more trustworthy than analytical philosophies. Berkeley had maintained that our knowledge of a material world rests on our senses; but our senses afford us *only* knowledge of our sensations or ideas; these sensations, however, do not correspond to any reality in the material world. Reid objects to the use of the word *only*, maintaining that such a view deprives the world around us of reality and makes of it an appearance, a dream. Reid's argument (anticipating some aspects of the phenomenological method of thinking) goes as follows: just as the power of art over the material world is limited to the connection and separation of already existent matter, it being unable to create new matter, so thought does not "produce" the outside world. Knowledge does not originate in sensations or ideas; it exists objectively in nature. The material world is not a dream but a reality.[4]

Common sense, as applied by Rosenzweig, neither utilizes preconceptions nor moves towards prearranged goals and "postulates." Not even God is "given" in advance of actual experience. During the period Rosenzweig worked on this small book, he wrote to his mother: "The chief thing is not whether a person 'believes' in the good Lord; what matters is that he open all his five senses and sees the facts—at the risk that even the good Lord may be found among the facts."[5]

Adherence to experience and common sense does not guarantee success. Terms are only vaguely defined and may mean different things to different people. (Both Hume and Berkeley professed to follow the principles of common sense!) One is reminded of a story told by the scientist Karl Compton. A sister who lived in India had a wiring job done by a native electrician who returned to her several times for instructions. Finally, the exasperated lady said: "You know very well

what I want. Why don't you use your common sense and go ahead?"
The electrician bowed gravely and replied: "Madame, I have only a
technical education. Common sense is a rare gift of God."

III

Chapter Two of *Understanding the Sick and the Healthy* offers a
contemptuous criticism of the "as if" philosophy represented by Hans
Vaihinger and his book *Philosophie des Als-Ob* which appeared in
1911. This construction, which goes back to Kant and to ideas expressed
by Friedrich Carl Forberg (1770-1848) maintains the following:
There is no God. A belief in God is, therefore, meaningless. Yet this
does not imply that religion should be abandoned. Religion, after all, is
more than a belief in God. It is a form of conduct based on such a belief.
To achieve this practical end it does not matter whether God is a reality
or an imaginary being. It is sufficient to accept the fiction of a god. In
theory I may know that God does not exist; in practice, however, I act
as if God did exist, as if I were responsible to him. Thus, religion is
understood as an organization of human behavior based on a theological fiction.

Invoking Kant's critical philosophy, Vaihinger interprets the statement "I believe in God" to mean: I act as if the existence of God were
a reality. My theoretical reason prohibits me from accepting a moral
law, but I act as if such a moral law existed because my practical reason
commands me to do the good absolutely. . . . Thus also the theoretical
atheist who acts in accordance with ethics "believes in God"—practically.[6] Such an approach to religion Vaihinger detects even in such an
ardent Christian as Schleiermacher. As a philosopher Schleiermacher
cannot perceive a relationship between God and the world; as a theo-
logian he assumes such a relationship as analogous to a father relationship to his child. This means: God is not the father of mankind, but he
should be treated as if he were.[7]

Not only God becomes a victim of the "as if" fiction. Man's freedom
is also a fiction. We are to consider man as if he were free. But he is not
free. All our perception is based on our will; our thinking produces these
ideas because they serve our purposes, because we need them. "Truth is
no longer ours," as Nietzsche has said.

Rosenzweig, in contrast to Vaihinger, considers man as a whole whose reason is not divided into a theoretical and a practical aspect. He cannot believe therefore that the "as if" approach can bring man "inner and outer peace."[8] Far from being able to cure the invalid the notion of "as if" can only add to his confusion.

The human patient, paralyzed by philosophy—of which the "as if" theory is only one example—is cured once he has learned to understand world, men and God as primary forms which underly reality. According to Rosenzweig, the same experience which leads to perception of the world, man and God, opens the vision of how they relate as well. For these relationships Rosenzweig chose terms from the realm of religion: Creation—Revelation—Redemption. The presentation of these relationships in their historical formulations (Judaism and Christianity) and in their significance for the life of the individual is contained in *The Star of Redemption*. But the patient who has overcome his paralysis and learned to walk again will put his legs to good service and walk in the right direction.

Several contemporary writers accord Rosenzweig a place among the existentialists. Though this may help his reputation in some circles it in no way advances the understanding of his works. True, the starting point of his thinking coincides with existentialism: the lonely, suffering individual, aware of his mortality—the human creature whose existence precedes thought. Rosenzweig frees the individual from his isolation; in relating himself to his fellow-man, to the world around him and to God, man's life becomes meaningful. His individual soul, unique and irreducible, participates in the dialogue with the other elements which constitute reality. Thus man's existence is truly co-existence. And if the reader desires an "ism" to cover Rosenzweig's thought, then, for argument's sake, it may be termed co-existentialism.

IV

In contrast to the traditional, abstract, "logical" thinking, Rosenzweig, following a theory of Eugen Rosenstock Huessy, calls the new method "grammatical thinking." Here human language, communication, the word, the name, are signs of reality, even keys to the understanding of reality. The problem of language and the name is an old one. In Plato's *Cratylus* the question is raised whether through an understanding of names we may be led to a knowledge of things. Hermogenes denies any relationship between name and reality; whereas Socrates insists on a deep connection between the existent thing and its name as a basis for our knowledge of reality. Plato, however, abandoned the position of this dialogue in the *Seventh Epistle*. Here the whole realm of language is taken to be only the first step to knowledge. The word strives to name true being but it cannot; ultimately, instead of expressing reality, the word becomes a barrier between the speaking person and the one spoken to. The thinker is left alone, to struggle in silence with the paradox of name, word and language.[9]

The two lines of thought, indicated by the *Cratylus* and the *Seventh Epistle* are continued through the Middle Ages. The "realism" of the Middle Ages (supported by Aristotelian logic which was grounded upon language) cultivated the word; its "nominalism" perpetuated the Sophists' scepticism of the word. The reality of language, "the force and signification of words," appeared as a problem at least to most modern philosophers. The great defender of language was Wilhelm von Humboldt, who perceived the interdependence of speech and cognition, and recognized that the word was not only an expression of reality but also a means by which to explore it. Hegel also believed that language possessed the power to express reality. But in the case of Hegel it becomes clear that language is primarily conceptual terminology and the word primarily an element of definition. The view of the French traditionalist V. G. A. de Bonald, may be of some interest. De Bonald questioned the value of autonomous reason and argued that the root of both reason and the intellectual life was grounded in language. The word, he maintained, comes to man as a divine revelation. It is the source of all truth; man's thought participates in it, but does not create it. The authoritative representation of this truth is to be found in the Church, which teaches the universal reason. De Bonald knew that language is more than a technical instrument, but theological dogmatism and vagueness led him astray; from beneath his religious theory shines Hegel's idea of the Objective Spirit.

The more recent trends in philosophy move towards ever greater distrust of language. Bertrand Russell *(The Scientific Outlook)* sees in language a collection of abstract nouns expressing an atomized universe of sense data. It is a language which can no longer serve as a means of communication between men. Here we may discover, in the words of W. M. Urban, "a progressive paralysis of speech." To Henri Bergson *(Creative Evolution, Introduction to Metaphysics)* language, being "static," cannot express the dynamic continuity of reality. Language is wedded to intellect and logic; reality can be fathomed only by immediate intuition which is non-logical, wordless. Here, too, speech is paralyzed. That language does violence to immediate experience is the conviction of A. N. Whitehead *(Process and Reality)*. He, therefore, wishes to redesign language and create a new system of categories of speech. Our universe, being a universe of "events" and "activity," would be adequately expressed in a language of verbs. As there are "no things," no names can be uttered to designate them.[10] Such speech, however, possibly considered "adequate" by philosophers (who, as Bertrand Russell says, "as a rule believe themselves free from linguistic forms") will never reach the ear of a living and speaking human being.

All this points to an abyss between man and the world beyond man. Nietzsche felt this incompatibility keenly and was thus able to allude to its root. "That world is well hidden from man! . . . that heavenly nothingness! The bosom of Being does not speak to man, except in the guise of man. Truly, all being is difficult to prove; it is difficult to make it speak."[11] Man's isolation from the world of Being, from the world outside the confines of the individual is at the root of this tragic silence. In Sartre's words, "there is no sign in the world." The names are dormant and man cannot invoke them. Man can think and create terminologies and classifications—outside of language and outside of time.

Against this background, Rosenzweig's New Thinking restores the relationship between man and world and God and with it the trust in man's power to speak and to communicate. Since, as Hölderlin tells us, "we exist as talk, and can hear from one another," we *do* speak and *do* listen. *Understanding the Sick and the Healthy* describes in three bold movements the role of language, the word and the name, in man's relation to the three elements which form reality. To Rosenzweig, language is not the "essence" of the world; it is "a bridge between the world and other things": God and the Self. And the name calls the Self into its presence.

In a later essay, Rosenzweig summarizes his teaching as contrasted to earlier modes of thinking. In the New Thinking, he says, the *method of speech* replaces the method of abstract, pure, timeless thinking maintained in earlier philosophies. Speech, on the other hand, is bound to time and nourished by time. It takes its cue from others. It lives by virtue of the life of the other person. Abstract thinking is always a solitary affair, even if it is done by several who philosophize together. For in that case, the other is only raising the objections I should raise myself. In a real dialogue an action takes place. I do not know in advance what the other person will say to me. The abstract thinker knows his thoughts in advance. The "speaking thinker" cannot anticipate anything; he must be able to wait because he depends on the word of the other; he requires *time*. The abstract thinker thinks for no one else and speaks to no one else. The "speaking thinker" speaks to someone and thinks for someone; a someone who has not only ears but also a mouth.[12]

V

The Star of Redemption, the fundamental document of the New Thinking, contains a lengthy discourse on Judaism and Christianity as historical realities. It does not attempt to prove that one is better than the other; nevertheless, once the book had been completed, its author was convinced that he had written a Jewish book.

The present treatise arrives at an understanding of Man—World—God as factors of reality. There is no effort to demonstrate the historic, philosophical, or religious forms in which this reality would be mirrored or manifested. Yet the *Lehrhaus* lectures in which Rosenzweig outlined the common sense view of *Understanding the Sick and the Healthy* were announced under the title: "A Guide to Jewish Thinking."

Such a name for a course which obviously had "nothing to do" with Jewish issues calls for an explanation. A chance remark, made shortly after the writing of the present book, gives an important insight into Rosenzweig's method of working. Stating that he is just as little an "expert" in Judaica as is Max Weber, Rosenzweig added: "The Jewish way [*das Jüdische*] is not my object but my method."[13] *Jewish,* in

Rosenzweig's estimation, is the insistence on the concrete situation; the importance of the spoken word and the dialogue; the experience of time and its rhythm and, in connection with it, the ability to wait; finally, the profound significance of the name, human and divine.

These elements and others contribute towards a *method* of thinking. Equally they become to Rosenzweig the means of expressing his thought. He uses the ancient words of classical Judaism, because, as he says, he has received the New Thinking in these ancient words. "I know that instead of these, New Testament words would have risen to a Christian's lips. But these were the words that came to me. And I really believe that this [*The Star of Redemption*] is a Jewish book; not merely one that treats of 'Jewish matters' . . . but a book of which the old Jewish words have formed the expression of whatever it has to say, and especially of what is new in it. Jewish matters are always past, as is matter generally, but Jewish words, however old, partake of the eternal youth of the word."[14]

VI

At about the same time that Rosenzweig was writing *Understanding the Sick and the Healthy,* Franz Kafka was working on *The Castle.* In this work a land surveyor, K, receives a call to do work in a castle; he arrives at the village which is dominated by the castle, only to find out that the castle is inaccessible to him, that even the lowest officials cannot be reached, and that his claim to having received a call cannot be verified. The villagers, who live without asking questions, and are protected by a naive sense of security, regard K as a stranger: "We do not need a surveyor; the boundaries of our small holdings are well marked out." K remains isolated from both castle and village; his knowledge estranges him from the simple village folk that do not know; but he cannot translate this knowledge into life, because real, meaningful, eternal life is in the castle and beyond the reach of knowing man. Man's tragic situation results from having eaten from the tree of knowledge and not having eaten from the tree of life.[15] "We are separated from God from both sides: the tree of knowledge separates us from Him, the tree of life separates Him from us."[16] With the expulsion from Paradise man lost his name (Kafka's heroes go mainly by initials), lost his language (there is no real communication), lost his love (only sex remains); time which could now be man's is but confused, distorted, paralyzed eternity. Man (K), World (village) and God (castle) exist, but their existences are not correlated.

Rosenzweig realized that Kafka was dealing with a genuinely biblical problem and said: "I have never read a book that reminded me so much of the Bible as *The Castle*."[17] Rosenzweig meets man exactly where Kafka had left him. To the biblical question of Kafka, the existentialist novelist, Rosenzweig, the co-existentialist thinker, gives the biblical answer, for he admits the biblical idea of Revelation (love). Thus man finds his place *next* to his fellow man, *in* the world and *before* God. He speaks and he is spoken to. He is called by his name and he names beings around him. And he has overcome his distrust of time; he has learned to wait (man was driven out of paradise because of impatience, says Kafka) until he "perceives in proper time," until time itself becomes a mirror of eternity.

VII

Rosenzweig, who regarded with suspicion all philosophical theories, programs, systems, speculations, doubted the validity of his own view—unless it could be verified in actual life. *The Star of Redemption* appeared to Rosenzweig to be "only a book." He did "not attach any undue importance to it." "The book is no goal, not even a provisional one."[18] The present work was not to his liking and therefore dropped. *The Star* had concluded with the words: Into life. That was what Rosenzweig called *no-more-book*. As a statement it could be accepted, rejected, criticized or derided like any other statement. In itself it is not "true." The present treatise concludes with a view of death as the brother of life. This statement is not "true" in itself. The verification can take place only in the midst of real life. Only here, in life, does it become clear whether we are faced by what Henry James called "the platitude of mere statement" or—by something different.

A note written by Rosenzweig to a poem of Judah ha-Levi explains what he meant. "Had Luther died on the thirtieth of October, 1517, all the audacity of his commentary on the 'Epistle to the Romans' would have been nothing but the extravaganzas of a late scholastic." But on the thirty-first Luther had nailed to the church door at Wittenberg his revolutionary ninety-five theses. Thus "life complemented the theory and made it true."[19]

Here a curious parallel comes to mind in the words of another critic of Hegelian philosophy: William James. Of truth he says: "Truth *happens* to an idea. It *becomes* true, is *made* true by events. Its verity is in fact an event, a process: the process namely of its verifying itself, its veri-*fication*. Its validity is the process of its valid*ation*."[20]

In comparing Kierkegaard with the modern theologians Karl Barth and Friedrich Gogarten, Rosenzweig finds that "behind each paradox of Kierkegaard one senses biographical *absurda,* and for this reason one must *credere.* While behind Barth's colossal negations one senses nothing but the wall on which they are painted, a whitewash wall, his immaculate and well-ordered life. . . . Not that they are unbelievable; but it is, after all, an indifferent authenticity."[21]

This treatise, too, would have remained a mere program. But even though it was not written out of an inner necessity, it was converted into a testimony by the subsequent life of its author. In the eight years until his death at forty-three, Rosenzweig had verified under the most tragic circumstances what he had professed in this book: a victory over the "nothings" that threaten man's freedom to think and to act; an affirmation of the three factors—God, world, man—whose relationships constitute reality; a passionate devotion to human language; a love of life and an acceptance of death. Rosenzweig's reflections can be contradicted; his life cannot.

Understanding the Sick and the Healthy is being printed and offered to the public not primarily as "a contribution to contemporary philosophical or religious thought," but as a part of Franz Rosenzweig's very life.

N. N. G.

Dear Sir:

I have decided reluctantly to release this little book, since I knew I would be unable to prevent it from reaching your hands.

And you will pick it up just as you, and others like you, pick up a book which confesses from the very beginning that it is addressed to everyone. You would of course permit me to address myself, in popular language, to the "masses," allowing them, in their way, to partake of the thoughts conceived in the quiet of the study. However, this little book is meant for everyone, including you, dear Sir. Yet we can hardly expect you to condescend to such an inclusion. On the contrary, your strongest confidence and self-assurance comes from the certainty that no one will dare to think of you when the simple word "everyone" is uttered.

Therefore, you will be quick, I know, to unsheathe that awe-inspiring weapon, the term "unscientific," eager for the kill. Behold—here is the chance to fulminate anathema. I cannot, and what is more, am unwilling to dodge the thrust.

I am in the pleasant position of being able to place my Introduction at the very end of the finished work. Although this puts me at a disadvantage with regard to you, the situation holds some rewards for me. The work itself is scientific, in its rounded shape and its inclusiveness, self-sufficient. An introduction can only introduce—in itself, it is not scientific. Anyone in quest of proof will be disappointed by it, and it will be of no help to him who has gone beyond the desire to question.

An introduction introduces and that is all it offers in the way of proof. It cannot, of necessity, be conclusive. An introduction is not self-contained; the end to which it points serves as final verification. The *end* validates the beginning.[22]

But all of this is a digression. You cannot possibly agree with it; you cannot even understand me, since you are what you cannot fail to be: the "expert." How can I dare to hope that you will cease to be that, and change into the man I shall now perforce address: the reader.

Here, Sir, standing on the threshold, I bid you goodbye.

Remaining *a limine* in everything,

Respectfully,

Your Author.

My very dear friend,

By now, I may assume, you are accustomed to such intimate address. The presumptious, backslapping manner of philosophers peddling a pretentious metaphysics is crude indeed. One should not attempt to force familiarity after a brief acquaintance. Accordingly I, for one, will try not to offend against good taste. Yet I do not wish to approach you as a stranger, but as an old acquaintance.

Try to remember your school days. Classmates and friends, we attended school together for quite some time: our school, the school of common sense. The memory of those days is the only bond to which I lay claim. Since then we have passed through other schools and have entered life. Now our paths cross once more. I do not find it difficult to address you familiarly, because my recollections of that first school have again become so strong and vivid; it is as if my old schoolmates stand before me as they were then.

Naturally you are not at all sure that you care for the rapid pace I am setting. You would welcome more tact and restraint on my part. It will be to your advantage for me to forego tact.

By the time we part again I hope the memory of our student days will have become so vivid for you that you will once more recognize
Your Author,
Who now, on the threshold, bids you a friendly welcome.

CHAPTER **1** *The Attack of Paralysis*

Common sense is in disrepute with philosophers. Its usefulness is restricted to the buying of butter, the courtship of a lady, or it may even be of help in determining the guilt of a man accused of stealing. However, to decide what butter and woman and crime "essentially" [*eigentlich*] are, is beyond its scope.

This is where the philosopher must enter and assume "the burden of proof." Such problems are beyond the reach of common sense. These are the "highest" problems, the "ultimate" questions. To be misunderstood by common sense is the privilege, even the duty of philosophy. What need would there be for philosophy if common sense could answer these questions by itself? Is common sense even capable of asking the questions? Where common sense proceeds in reckless haste, philosophy pauses and wonders. And were it merely a question of this gift, alone, this capacity to wonder, philosophy's rightful claim to superiority could not be disputed. For common sense, as it is said, is not addicted to the ways of wonder.

But, be this as it may, how does our philosopher know of wonder? In any case, where does he obtain the word? Does not the non-philosophizing half of mankind also wonder? The wonder of a child? The wonder of the savage? Does not wonder overcome them a hundred times—even oftener than the philosopher? True, the continuity of life blunts the edge of marvelling. Wonder is finally enveloped in the stream of time. It vanishes as naturally as it appeared.

The child wonders at the mature man. The quest, however, which is at the core of his wonder, is painlessly fulfilled when the child grows into a mature man.

Woman is aroused by man and man submits to woman. But even as they marvel at each other the solution and dissolution of their wonder is at hand—the love which has befallen them. They are no longer a wonder to each other; they are in the very heart of wonder.

Life becomes numb in the face of death—and dies. The wonder is unraveled. And it was life itself that brought the solution.

Thus man wonders. Undoubtedly he pauses—to wonder requires that man pause.[23] He pauses but he cannot remain still. He is adrift on the river Life, borne on, wonderment and all. He merely drifts and goes on living, and then, at last, the numbness caused by his wonder passes. But drifting, alas, does not become the wondering philosopher.

The philosopher cannot wait. His kind of wonder does not differ from the wonder of others. However, he is unwilling to accept the process of life and the passing of the numbness wonder has brought. Such relief comes too slowly. He insists on a solution immediately—at the very instant of his being overcome—and at the very place wonder struck him. He stands quiet, motionless. He separates his experience of wonder from the continuous stream of life, isolating it.

This is the way his thought proceeds. He does not permit his wonder, stored as it is, to be released into the flow of life. He steps outside the continuity of life and consequently the continuity of thought is broken. And there he begins stubbornly to reflect. Of necessity, he must hook the "problem" from where he stands. He has forcibly extracted thought's "object" and "subject" from the flow of life and he entrenches himself within them. Wonder stagnates, is perpetuated in the motionless mirror of his meditation: that is in the subject. He has it well-hooked; it is securely fastened, and it persists in his benumbed immobility. The stream of life has been replaced by something submissive—statuesque, subjugated.

Entrenched within the subject, the philosopher asks: what then actually *is?* He welcomes any answer which does not destroy the value and meaning of this single question. Remove this immovable question and the lifeless subject, artificially detached, must inevitably disappear.

His question is: what actually *is?* It is a stubborn question and now it takes vengeance on him. To refuse stubbornly to wait with patience is to surrender life. He receives as his reward one unfailing answer, always the same. Asking, as he does, outside the full expanse of life, not waiting for a leisurely answer, he must ask his questions there and then —and there and then the answers are given.

They cannot come in their own time, and therefore they are lacking in extension and completeness. Driven to subterranean regions, the answers rise from beneath the surface of the subject—that is, from its sub-stance.[24] The true concern of the philosopher is with the "essence," the "essential" being of his subjects. He does not have to wait for an answer to his question. Answers wait for him in eager readiness, as independent of time and its processes as is the subject, which also has been detached from the stream of life by means of an artificial fixative: the timeless artificiality of the question "what actually *is.*" The question receives its answer: "the essence." This answer may not sound unnatural, and indeed it is the only possible answer, once the unnatural question is asked.

Necessarily there can be only one *substantial* mark setting apart the multiplicity of things. What else is there in *reality* to make us realize that this act is our act? Precisely the experience of such an act as a consequence of our past life and an anticipation of the future as its outcome! A thing receives a character of its own only within the flow of life. The question, "what is this actually?", detached from time, deprived of it, quickly passes through the intermediary stage of the general term and comes into the pale region of the mere "thing." Thus emerges the concept of the one and only substance, the "essential" nature of things. The singleness and particularity [*Eigenheit*] of the subject detached from time is transformed into a statement of its particular essence [*Eigentlichkeit des Wesens*].

"Essential" [*eigentlich*]—no one but a philosopher asks this question or gives this answer. In life the question is invalid; it is never asked. Indeed, even the philosopher, when the situation becomes serious, refrains from asking it. He is scarcely interested in knowing what half a pound of butter costs "essentially." He does not court his beloved in proper terms of essence. He would neither deny nor affirm that the defendant stole, or did not steal, "essentially." The terms of life are not "essential" but "real"; they concern not "essence" but "fact." In spite of this, the philosopher's word remains, "essential." By giving in to wonder, by halting in his tracks and neglecting the operations of reality, he forces himself into retreat and is restricted to facing essence.

It is exactly at this point—not later—that the philosopher parts company with ordinary common sense. Common sense puts its faith in the strength of reality. The philosopher, suspicious, retreats from the flow of reality into the protected circle of his wonder; slowly he submerges to the depths, to the region of the essences. Nothing can disturb him there. He is safe. Why should he concern himself with the crowd of "non-essences." And reality, is, so to speak, "unessential." Bounded by his magic circle of mounting wonder, he is not interested in the actual event [*Ereignis*]. Should the actual event find entrance to the magic circle, it may be marvelled at—so much is allowed. However, it definitely may not destroy the immobility caused by wonder, nor let loose the damned-up tide. It may not stir up the storm of life—existing as yet only in strings of essences—and permit it to sweep through the sturdy forests of reality.

If this were merely some philosopher's personal concern, we would not object; there are so few philosophers, even taking into account the assorted breeds. But as it happens, any man can trip over himself and find himself following the trail of philosophy. No man is so healthy as to be immune from an attack of this disease. And the very moment a man succumbs, the instant he believes that philosophizing is necessary, he gives up common sense, and the ardor of his quest in search of essence cannot be surpassed. Then the wisest man is no match for him; with ease he outdoes professional philosophers. No one has less faith in himself than he. Common sense is crippled by a stroke. We shall view it in this state of utter paralysis.

2 CHAPTER *Visit at the Sickbed*

We approach our bedridden patient. He was forced to take to his bed; suddenly he was unable to attend to even the most urgent necessities of daily life. He is paralyzed: numbed by wonder. His hands will not grasp—they await some justification to act. His legs refuse to move—how can they be sure the ground is solid? His eyes refuse to see—what proof is there that everything is not a dream? And as for his ears, they refuse to hear—to whom should they listen? His mouth is closed in silence; talk in empty space is of little use.

What has happened to him? Yesterday he walked, happy and untroubled enjoying the fruit of the trees that lined his way, exchanging friendly words with comrades on his journey. Then suddenly bewilderment seized him and confined him to a darkened sickroom; he put stoppers in his ears and refused to permit a soul near him.

The troubled relatives, distraught with worry, hastily summoned a famous healer who peddles infallible medicines on street corners. This man put on his omniscient mien: "The reason for your ailment is quite obvious—we will apply an unfailing remedy. You say you doubt the aim of life. A matter of no consequence, try to forget it; just act as if the aim still existed."[25]

"But, after all, I am not sure it does exist."

"Never mind that, never mind—what you have to do is to talk yourself into certainty. By daily, nay, by hourly exercise you must reinforce your system of 'as if' and success will not be long in coming."

"Tell me, do you believe in it yourself?"

"That's quite unnecessary, dear man. Nor do I expect you to believe it. Just act as if you did believe. I'll guarantee the results. You can depend on that. At least pretend that you depend on it."

"But even if I did, I am unsure of more than life's purpose; the road I am traveling, my very acts, have become uncertain. I do not know whether it is I who acts. I do not know whether it is I who am acted upon. I am not certain that what is occurring is not merely a dream of acting and enduring."

"That unfortunately is a further complication. However, our well-established treatment is capable of handling it. A thorough application is required. Now, then, simply pretend that you do pretend."

"Do I understand you to say that I must pretend that I pretend to act? Sir—"

"Don't talk back. As if! As if! You wish absolute certainty. The treatment, however, has been thoroughly tested. The departments of philosophy, law, medicine, and happily, even that of theology, have approved it.[26] It has been recommended by the leading minds of our universities and colleges. Actually the treatment was invented forty years ago—but only very recently did the inventor decide to benefit the public at large by its disclosure.[27] It is a synthesis of simplified Kant and stultified Nietzsche. Really it's childishly easy to understand and apply. Of course you are not a child any longer; that much is presupposed. You wish to buy a pound of butter and discover that you have forgotten your purse —a simple matter: act as if you were paying. You'll see; the cashier will be completely satisfied. You want to marry? Just pretend you are married. It is a good deal cheaper and it comes to the same thing. You are a member of a jury and you hesitate to pronounce a man guilty because you have qualms about capital punishment. A problem of no consequence: why not pretend to execute the man? It makes no difference to you and certainly he will not object. 'Consider yourself re-

44

proved,' may have sounded shallow once; today it has become meaningful. As if this were not a measure of progress!"

"Forgive my interrupting, but it seems as if I understand. What you are saying is simply that, since I have lost assurance of life's purpose, as well as its direction and reality, I should pretend that it has purpose; I should act as if what I called *my* purpose was really a purpose—well, perhaps. How can I act, however, how can I pretend when I am no more certain about 'I' than about the ways and purposes of the external world? However much I may be willing to accept 'as if,' responsibility for action and the end of action requires an actor, and I, the actor, am uncertain of myself."

"An actor? You have not grasped the half of it! We can do without an actor. Merely substitute 'as if' for the actor, and the circle is closed. If you are uncertain of yourself, just proceed. I have no more certainty than you. Of course, you must act as if *you* were acting—you continually. The last link in the chain has been snapped into its proper place. God, world, you yourself, all that is, are woven into one great 'as if.' There is only one way to exist: be as if you were. That covers everything. It is the all-containing cellar underlying reality. It is essentially. . ."

"Sir, it is already dark enough. There is no need to lead me to additional cellars. I urgently desire to be helped from, not locked into, the cellar."

"Dear Sir, you seem to forget I am a philosopher. Duty leads me to the cellar."

"That's unfortunate for you. As for me, I want to get out of the cellar."

"Sir, do you want to be cured or not?"

"Will you be satisfied if I say that it is as if I wanted to be cured?"

"Preposterous. I did not come here to be ridiculed."

The patient does not answer.

The famous practitioner departs. The patient's hopes have reached a low ebb; his distrust has grown. What can we possibly offer now? We begin by cautiously questioning him about the early period of his illness; and we are told that nothing of particular significance occurred. He had gone about his duties as usual and then suddenly he had been struck by thought. He had stopped, and, when he wanted to continue, he had found himself unable to do so. The very ground beneath him had been undermined. His own body seemed a stranger to him. He had not known how near or far objects were from him; the horizon had wavered. In short, all that he had taken for granted became uncertain; he had required proof and assurance of everything. Thus it was that he had stopped, that he was unable to proceed.

A most serious case. The diagnosis is simple. We take the patient's pulse as a matter of routine and find it to be slow, of course. He hasn't much temperature. The symptoms are what we had thought them to be, simple enough to interpret. Therapy, however, is a more difficult matter.

CHAPTER **3** *Diagnosis*

To clarify further the issue, the reader must permit me a chapter dealing with the physiology of the mind. As soon as he learns the symptoms of the illness, he will understand why this procedure is necessary.

How does common sense perform its task? Let us return to our example of the pound of butter. If we imagine the mental process of the buyer, we discover two possibilities: either he left home with the intention of buying or he decided to do so when he passed the shop. Both possibilities have one thing in common—the slab of butter he finally buys is a very definite slab. Now, when did it become that particular piece? The instant the man at the counter sliced it. Or, perhaps, even earlier. If the latter, it may have happened when he discovered the butter in the shop window. What had it been previous to this? Nothing. And if the buyer did set out from home with the intention of buying butter, was it only butter in general that he had in mind? Certainly not.

His intention of buying butter requires the memory of another, and very specific slab of butter, eaten by him, let us say, yesterday. Even in this instance, the general concept "butter" serves only as the intermittent link between the particular slab, the taste of which still lingers on his tongue, and the other particular slab which he finds in the grocery store. This intermittent link of "butter in itself" may be given, but the example of a sudden decision to buy shows that it does not have to exist. The assertion that it must exist, even in the latter case, is unfounded.

What is at the root of this assertion? An observation so simple it is scarcely worth mentioning. The butter remembered, the butter desired, and the butter finally bought, are not the same. They may even be quite different. But they are always a "something." It follows that some bond between them must exist. This idea—that of a connecting link—is closely bound up with the general concept of "butter in itself," which, as we have seen, sometimes does act as a connecting link.

Philosophy has claimed, since time immemorial, that the general concept is given, even if it is not perceptible. The "butter in itself" is the "idea" of butter; it is what the butter is "essentially." Actually, no one has ever seen this "ideal" butter which is always "present." On close inspection, it vanishes. It becomes only a subordinate line, attempting to connect two points: yesterday's butter and today's. Indeed, as it traversed this line, the butter did not resemble butter in general; it resembled yesterday's butter up to the moment when the buyer sighted the butter in the shop window—then it became today's butter. At some decisive point in its movement, the transition from yesterday to today took place. But indeed how? Is it really timelessness which mediates between two separate points in time?

What has actually taken place? I transform the representation of my wish, as yet resembling the image in my memory, into what I see in the shop window. If we consider the matter without prejudice, we observe that after this change has taken place, nothing but the word "butter" remains the same. Is this all, then, nothing but a mere word, a name? Yes, indeed, this is all, only a name. All else has changed; the name remains. This is the first fact that must be stated. And what do we gain by such a statement? Above all, we make certain that no one is tempted to assume that the name is the "essence" of the thing. No one can say that the word "butter" *is* butter. Indeed the word alone endures; it can be said of the word that it has been *and* is *and* will be. All else either has been, *or* is, *or* will be. Only the name was yesterday, is today, and will be tomorrow. The name, however, is not the thing which it

48

Diagnosis describes.[28]

A similar example is the courtship which precedes marriage. Time elapses between the decision to propose and the eventual consent or rejection. When it is a case of love at first sight, as, for instance, with Romeo and Juliet, the length of time may be considerably reduced. But then, on the other hand, time may drag on. War has been known to force a lapse of years between question and acceptance. Whatever the instance, time is required. And since time must elapse, the answer is unavoidably given by another person than the one who was asked, and it is given to one who has changed since he asked it. It is impossible to know how profound the change has been. Let us assume that it is insignificant. Nevertheless, a whole lifetime is involved in question and answer. The lovers dare not deny, not even Romeo and Juliet, that changes, involving both of them, will inevitably take place. Nevertheless they do not hesitate. Indeed, the man who proposes and the woman who replies do not reflect upon these vicissitudes. They cling to the unchangeable. What is the unchangeable? Unbiassed reflection reveals once more that it is only a name. In this instance, it is the names of the respective lovers. And appropriately enough, the first relief from tension in the enchanted game of love usually comes when the lovers call each other by their first names. This act stands as a solitary pledge that the yesterdays of the two individuals will be incorporated in their today.

Once more only names. Who will maintain that the lovers "are" their names? "What are you?" is the question involving existence; the question concerning essence remains unasked. It has been made superfluous by the implicit answer to an unspoken question. "Who are you?" is the question, and the reply is, "John." There is no need to formulate the question. It does manifest itself, however, disguised as a gnawing doubt, when lovers have been long separated: how can a person—any person —be so faithful to himself as to remain faithful to another? But as soon as the "person" becomes "John"—well-defined by his name—the doubt disappears. The name is not the "essence." Yet, although the name and the essence are not identical, the name is as permanent as the essence is supposed to be. And common sense in action is concerned that the name, not the "essence," remain.

A very similar instance is that of a trial. Let us assume that the guilt of the defendant has been ascertained. The offense was committed in the past, perhaps a long time previous. The sentence extends far into the future. The criminal may change between the date of his sentence and the beginning of his punishment; and it is practically certain he will change, for better or worse, during the period of his imprisonment. And in addition, so much time having elapsed, the attitude of the public toward the crime may change. It may come to be considered a more reprehensible act or, on the other hand, a negligible offense; it may even, as is often the case with political crimes, be looked upon as a deed of heroism. The sentence does not concern itself with these possibilities. The prevailing legal designation of the crime is all it needs to know. The offense has been given a name and this is the decisive factor. The sentence remains in force until the name of the crime is changed and an "outrageous act" is transformed—by a shift of opinion—into an "immortal deed."

So again the name is decisive. The act, however, is not identical with its classification. It would be absurd to maintain such a position. No act is simply a theft. It is as contingent and involved as it appears to the delving sympathy of a poet. The act is not identical with its classification, but it is judged according to its classification. Even if its features change completely, it remains what it has always been. The judgment remains until the name is changed. The name of the crime fuses act, trial, and sentence into a unity.

Of course, we must not overlook one important difference. In the two former instances, the name existed through general consent; here there is more than this, and this more must be considered. The judge is in part a legislator. He not only classifies an act by a given legal term, but, within limits, he decides as well what that act has been. What does this imply? Does he inquire about the "essence" of the act? We may rest assured that if he did he would share the poet's fate; he would uncover a multitude of aspects without ever decisively establishing the act as a crime, much less that particular crime. He merely assigns a legal name to the deed confronting him. This act of naming differs from the other two instances to this extent: here the name retains an element of variability. We stated that the word indicating the thing is not the thing itself, that John's name is not John. And now we discover that the classi-

50

fication is not the act which it classifies. Here again the designation is the immutable factor, although, in this case, only relatively immutable.

But it is understandable enough that common sense is, in this case, more easily confused than in the previous instances. And it is possible that we may gain important information about what happens in these other instances from its confusion here. What goes on in the mind of the judge? He is expected to pass judgment. Instead of doing this, he becomes involved in an insoluble problem: "Is there really such a thing as crime? I am the one who calls this highly complicated act a crime. There is no doubt that I find it complicated—and what is more, its meaning for others is changing continually; its meaning is changing even for the perpetrator himself. Is this act a crime? What is its essential character?"

The knowledge he has of his own part in classifying the act necessarily compels the judge to ask these questions. The more he reflects on it, the less certain he becomes of the end result, that is, of the classification of the act as a crime. Although it was he who called it a crime, he feels he might as easily have decided otherwise. And so he feels he cannot uphold the immutability of the classification; his confidence in the name is weakening. He seeks firmer ground, the actual situation, the facticity of the act, including its perpetrator. And thus he clamors for stability, for immutability and "essence," faced by a reality unwilling to yield him what he desires. Despairingly he asks: What is it actually?

Answers, of course, throng to him, beautifully theoretical answers about the essence of crime. None, however, pertain to this particular, concrete crime. At best they define crime in general, considering it to be sickness, sin, error, the result of social circumstances. Such answers may be of service, in their appropriate setting, to the physician, the priest, the teacher, or the statesman. To him, in his particular situation, they are worthless. He is the judge, he is to pronounce sentence. Inevitably he is thrown off-balance if he doubts the validity of the term which he must use in his official capacity. He can judge only if he preserves his faith in the particularity of the case presented to him for classification. However, the question, "What is it actually?" transforms the particular instance into "essence." The rest is silence—that is, for the judge at least. The stability of the term, the only tangible stability, has become suspect. And seeking for stability in things, he relegates them by his search to the dark realm of essence. These are the symptoms of one type of that illness with which we are becoming acquainted. The victims of this variety are legion.

The other two types are less frequent. Most people are likely to experience doubts about the possibility of reasonable action in the various fields of public life. By comparison, in the private life of a human being, the tendency to doubt is rare. It is even less frequent in the processes of cognition, that is, in the cognitive acts of everyday life. A queer fellow, indeed, who would refrain from marrying—to return again to our well-worn example—simply because he lacked confidence in himself and because he had no definite assurance of the love of the girl. Of course, the arguments he can advance are irrefutable. The attitude of "all in good time" can enable him to overcome his hesitation. But he does not adopt this attitude, because he insists on regarding the pertinent human data as isolated facts. A person in full possession of his common sense holds on to the names, the only tangible facts. This, however, does not relieve our fellow's doubts, since names are "arbitrarily" given by parents.

Now it becomes clear why this manner of thinking cannot be refuted. The lover merely applied the question "What actually is it?" to a human being. The answer he received resulted in the immediate disappearance of two very concrete individuals—the questioner himself and his beloved. No matter whether the answer is "the peak of creation" or "an insect crawling in the dust," the concrete individual is replaced by a ghost. The ghost may be of heaven or hell; it may be devil or angel—but a man cannot live with these rarified essences; and the question concerning the "essence" of man cannot yield more substantial results.

Sensible people consider a person sick who seeks such queer bypaths of thoughts. And, in this respect, the majority of mankind are sensible. The case we dealt with at the outset is even simpler, since it is purely theoretical. In practical life no one gives up his intention to buy butter merely because he is unable to prove that the butter he wishes to buy and the butter on sale are identical. The single exception to this is the

Diagnosis philosopher, but even he carefully restricts his meditations to theory. When he goes shopping he is unwilling to have an empty stomach as a reward for his thoughts. In theory, of course, he cannot be refuted. As soon as he asks: "What is this actually?" the butter disappears. As for the name—well, that is a matter of convention. Different languages have different names for one and the same thing. If a philosopher, however, should turn his back on our slab of butter, claiming it cannot be butter, because the French call it *beurre,* the proper place for him would be an institution accommodating philosophers exclusively.

We have used, as examples, cases which showed analogous symptoms. Our last example, a purely theoretical case, presented these symptoms without distortion; and we can assume that the symptoms we found here bear some resemblance to those found in real cases. In every instance the natural order of things is reversed. Common sense accepts the immutability of terms, be they words or personal names; it does not question the freedom of actions or things. However, the sick reason rejects names as worthless, and queries actions and things. "What are these actually?" it asks. The answer that it receives leaves everything in darkness, darkness which blurs all distinctions. There is no end here to doubt and despair. One is fortunate, if by a final effort of will, he is able to resist that panacea for doubt, the As-If cure. Should he have accepted it, his torments would only have increased. Now then, let us see what can be done.

CHAPTER **4** *Therapy*

What course of action must be chosen? Let us be warned by the bad example of indifferent physicians who believe that for a sickness, once it is recognized, there is but one possible therapy, effective under all circumstances. Such caution is particularly necessary if we are unable to localize the illness, and are convinced that the entire person, the complete individual, is affected. We must not insist on praising one particular treatment as a complete panacea when we have to deal with the affliction of a human being in his entirety. On the contrary, we are committed to considering a series of possible treatments, even though we run the risk that most of these treatments will prove unavailable to us.

As we have observed, our patient suffers from a radical inversion of his normal functions. It may be necessary to reverse the inversion, that is, turn matters upside-down. However, such a reversal, made arbitrarily, can prove dangerous. Man has a deep-rooted distaste for such "treatment." Common sense has already been inverted and become sick reason. Can a return to healthy common sense be forced?

Will such a forced return succeed? Experience answers in the affirmative. As it happens, all the phantoms of sick reason may be dissipated by a single event. A sudden fright, an unexpected happiness, a blow of fate beyond the ordinary can dispel at once all the delusions of the misdirected reason. Names take on again their original lustre—e.g., in August 1914 the word "fatherland" and all the theories of "essence" dissolved into nothing.

Of course, such a cure cannot be applied at will. To be effective, it must be part of living experience. Such a *tour de force* has another disadvantage; it does not heal permanently. Once the shock wears off, the man tends to return to what he considers his permanent condition. This "permanent" condition will most probably not be a normal state. We have every reason to believe that his constitution had deviated from normality, and was forced back only by the sudden shock. To make such a shock-cure last, milder and more enduring forces are necessary.

The appearance of such forces can well be expected. The sickness of reason is such an unusual condition, that it may be cured, at last, by the power of life itself. This is the well-known influence which "life" exerts on "ideals" and nothing is more feared by the sick reason than this influence. Everyday life, it is clear, cannot possibly be ignored; one cannot exist entirely in the sublime realm of theory, no matter how "essential" it may seem when compared to dull, tedious reality. The concerns of the world intrude. They bring with them the natural structure of life, the force of facts and experience, the impact of everyday existence with its interminable small tasks and its stable, enduring names. The revolutionary passion against names, permanent, traditional names, dies; the quest for a meaning, hidden behind events, ends; events come and go and no attempt is made to discover a meaning in them other than that revealed by the names by which they are called.

Is this, then, all there is to it? If so, then the return to common sense is identical with a return to philistinism—the natural concomitant of advancing age. However, something quite different happens. Common sense does return, it is true, but it remains unaware, as it were, of its return. It makes an effort to ignore this fact. Philistinism suffers from a sense of guilt. It knows exactly what it is—it knows it is habit and routine; however, it would prefer to be different. It is influenced in its self-evaluation by standards it rejects in practice but acknowledges in theory. Therefore, philistinism, although it is sane enough, finds itself in a worse situation than that which it has outgrown. The diseased life of the sick reason was lived in good faith; sick reason acted in accordance with its beliefs, that is, it believed nothing and did nothing. Philistinism, however, exists in health but is diseased in thought—to the extent that it thinks at all. It lives within time, for the day and its concerns, and believes in eternity, which is the name-less, transcendent nothing. It would be healthy if belief and action coincided. However, such is rarely the case. In the final analysis, a self-cure by means of time produces not true health but its travesty. What is generally produced by such a cure, is the philistine, and he can scarcely be considered a perfect specimen of health—rather the contrary.

An enticing therapeutical possibility presents itself at this point. The thought of the philistine is diseased, but his actions are healthy. Suppose we were to perform a major operation upon his thought, is it not possible that this might produce proper thinking? But unfortunately, surgery of this sort is of no help to us. Our enemy is not idealism as such; anti-idealism, irrationalism, realism, materialism, naturalism, and what not, are equally harmful. The real cause of the illness is not that reason assumes that "spirit" is the essence of reality; it is its assumption that it is possible for something to exist beyond reality. Reality, matter, nature, are all terms denoting "essence" and are just as unacceptable as "spirit" or "idea." All claim to "be" either reality itself or the "essence" of reality. All abstract from life. All neglect the fact of names. Consequently all these *isms* fail to conciliate thought and action, which is, after all, the one thing desired. They fail precisely because they are *isms,* whether "idealisms" or "realisms."

There is still another possibility, which, however, we must refrain from advocating too insistently, since it promises only a limited and conditional success. And furthermore, it cannot be denied that shock and time cures, treatments that do not require our active interference, may prove effective, although they are frequently, for the reasons mentioned, inoperative. Consequently this final treatment should be considered only as an additional possibility. It is particularly helpful if the patient has already begun his convalescence in time and experience.

One of the most powerful reasons why common sense becomes unbalanced and loses its self-confidence, is its alleged inability to answer the so-called "ultimate questions" concerning God, man, and the world. The syndrome we have been studying begins when the individual is struck dumb with wonder. Always it turns out that the wonderer was stricken just as he caught a glimpse, through rising clouds, of gigantic mountain peaks. The road of life winds among three mountain ranges, and, as is to be expected, they may be seen from many a bend in the road. That wanderer is lost who feels compelled to pause at such a point. The stopovers we viewed in the previous chapter were of this kind; they were a marvelling at distant vistas. Confidence in words, in the name of the beloved, in the designation of butter, in the legal appellation of a crime, were lost. To the faltering observer, unable to regard such matters as constituitive aspects of worldly existence, human destiny, or divine activity, the meaning of such terms has become uncertain.

Our task is to strengthen the reason, build up its weakened resistance at these three points. Since it has already become ill, it is necessary to relieve reason of its professional activities, as it were, and prescribe the isolation of a sanatorium. There we will attempt gradually to accustom it to these primary vistas [*Urgesichte*]. We are perfectly aware that such a treatment can have only limited success, and is feasible only to the degree that such encounters can be artificially arranged. The sole task of the physician is to help the patient get on his feet again after such encounters; it may even be limited to encouraging the patient not to stop. We are aware of our limitations and of the limitations of medicine in general. After a careful reading of the following chapter, the discriminating reader will be in a position to confirm our statement.

CHAPTER **5** *A Professional Exchange of Letters*

So that our reader will be able to understand what follows, we are making public a letter, addressed to the medical director of the sanatorium, and we print his reply.

Here is our letter:

Dear Sir:

You are, I know, well acquainted with the general features of a case I am referring to your institution in the near future. All the distinctive symptoms of acute *apoplexia philosophica* are to be found in it. Word has recently been going the rounds concerning certain outstanding therapeutic successes at your institution and, understandably enough, old practitioner that I am, I immediately recalled what I had heard as soon as the case was brought to my attention. I hope you will not object to my asking a question on this occasion. My professional curiosity is piqued by your ability to overcome those obstacles which generally confront one in the treatment of such cases.

Since the Criticin-vaccination[29] has been held in such high esteem for so many years, and has wrecked so many generations of patients, despite illusory successes in the first stages of treatment, it is fortunate that, at last, its disastrous consequences have come to be generally known. As you are, of course, aware, the expected reaction has set in. There is an attempt to mend one mistake by making another. It seems reasonable to assume that we will presently witness a craze for Mysticol injections of as universal a scope as the previous fad.

I am sure, dear Sir, that you agree that this treatment, as well as any treatment that subjects the human organism to entirely artificial conditions, should, except in a few very special cases, be rejected. We both know that a sick reason can only be cured if it is restored—by an application of some force, if necessary—to its normal environment. The task is not to "infuse" the patient's reason with something new, but to return it to the condition from which it deviated. We must fight the various mountebank cures, the ointments, the vaccinations, old or new, with the slogan "Environmental treatment." I can tell by a glance at the map that even the location of your sanatorium, equidistant from the three primary mountains,[30] offers enormous advantages for this kind of treatment.

One point, however, is unclear to my colleagues and me. How do you insure the patient a view of the peaks, since they are so often covered with clouds, and how do you prevent him from stubbornly staring at whichever peak happens to be visible at the moment? This is what we observe happens at the onset of the illness. There has been talk in professional circles about a revolving chair which mechanically produces a change of view; such a chair, it is thought, might counteract the tendency towards staring. Experimental verification of this treatment has been prevented by the fact that the three peaks in question, because of the unfavorable location of our town, cannot be seen clearly at the same time. However, it seemed to us that the more advantageous climactic conditions, along with the higher altitude of your establishment, might permit such a solution, or one very similar.

A clarification of these matters would add greatly to the knowledge of my colleagues and me. I sincerely apologize for the unexpected length of this letter; I fear that at times it very nearly became a treatise itself.

Very truly yours, etc., etc.

With the kind permission of the author, I publish his reply.

Dear Sir:

You were not mistaken in assuming that we share the same scientific attitude. I concur in your repudiation of the injection fad. However, a revolving chair is not a part of our method. In arriving at our method, we encountered the same obstacles of which you complain. The climactic conditions here are more or less the same as in your town; and so it would be impossible for us to keep the three peaks visible to the patient, alternating the view artificially. The method of which you have heard, and to which we owe our success, is considerably more primitive than you think. (We are aware of its limitations, and are hesitant to ascribe success exclusively to it.) Basically, at least it is an "Environmental" cure, if I may borrow your term. The location of the building is actually the main factor. Our building is at the precise geometrical center of the three ranges; there is the entire secret.

When I commenced building, several years ago, I made use of whatever roads and pathways I found. From a glance at the map you will see that roads lead from the building to all three ranges. The roads communicate with each other by byways even at their beginnings. Such byways, however, we do not consider. Nor do we concern ourselves with the incredibly complicated system of roads and pathways which have been created over the centuries. All of these roads finally terminate in a single highway which alone leads to the summit and which, what with attempts ending in accident and death, may have been traversed successfully no more than once.

I discovered that the confusion of roads and bypaths have a pattern, and that the routes to the various peaks are similar. For our purposes, this is a great asset, although it should be pointed out that to uncover the design it was necessary to employ a selective principle—and this was none other than expediency. Indeed some restrictive principle was necessary since there are such an incredible number of roads crossing the mountains. My choice of a "typical road" was justified by the therapeutic purpose it was to serve. However, it should be understood that alternate routes may prove equally useful. For instance, the route I used, and which I shall presently describe, is certainly not the most suitable for healthy climbers. They will, and should, continue to select routes fitted to their needs and desires even though these are more dangerous. The benefits to the community and to the health of the individual of an uninhibited zest for mountain climbing cannot be over-estimated. On the other hand, my simplified procedure proves to be highly effective for persons who are not in the best of health. Let me give you a provisional description of those elements of the treatment which are standard for all three cases.

In the complete darkness before sunrise, we transport the patient to the foot of the mountain by the shortest route. At daybreak he has a view of the foothills—no more. The entire massif is encircled by a road which rises slightly. The summit cannot be seen; however, as soon as the clouds lift, the peaks of the two other mountains become visible. Inevitably, of course, as the road curves, the view of one of the mountains is obscured. For one-third of the route it cannot be seen; on the next third the other mountain is not visible. The final third of the road curves away from the two peaks; this is the blind side of the mountain.

Though our patient is deprived of a panorama, this is compensated for by a close-up of enchanting beauty. Above him the massif rises to its towering summit, even the minutest detail visible to him in the piercing clarity of the alpine morning. Pardon my poetic raptures! My patients, it should be observed, are also overcome by enthusiasm. At a point where the road makes a full turn, the summit comes into view. From there on, the road winds continually so that much the same effect is gained as would be from your revolving chair; the view is constantly shifting from peak to peak. At the precise instant that the patient reaches the top, the entire panorama is revealed to him, both the summit he has ascended and the two peaks in the distance. Should there be a break in the clouds at this moment, he will also see beneath him a segment, sometimes large, sometimes small, of the familiar valley. This happens quite often, whereas the opposite—that is, an opportunity to view the three peaks simultaneously from the valley—is very rare. Thus our patient, viewing familiar territory, the commonplace and ordinary, at the same time that he reaches the summits, is oriented again. Actually his loss of orientation was the result of his sickness; it did not in my opinion provoke it. However, it can be fatal.

I hope that I have given a clear account of our treatment. The reports of our patient will add color to the diagram I have drawn for you. These reports are usually written by the patient himself during the week of rest which follows each stage of the cure. They are, I believe, an important part of the treatment, therapeutic in themselves, in addition to indicating the effect of the cure. I advise you to notice when you read the reports how the type of language used by the patient constantly changes. This is causally related to the change in the means of transportation used; the first trip is made by carriage, the second on horseback, and the last, if possible, on foot. If I can trust our previous experience, you will see evidence in the reports of your patient's increasing independence.

With best regards to you and your colleagues, I am sincerely

etc. etc.

So much for the letter. Now the patient begins his journey. In the following pages we shall reproduce the weekly reports the patient wrote at the sanatorium, at first entirely for his own use.

CHAPTER 6 *The Cure: First Week*

Nowadays a *Weltanschauung* is a valuable asset, and it would appear quite natural and obvious that the world should be "viewed."[81] However, the truth of the matter is that man becomes acquainted merely with certain fragments of the world at best coming in contact with only a limited number of things and people and events. If such a loose agglomeration of accidentally encountered fragments is considered the world, no harm need result from having a *Weltanschauung*. The word *Weltanschauung* is, however, sometimes associated with a much less modest claim. Here the word signifies more than a mere river bed passively permitting the stream of things and people and events to flow by; it is understood as a bowl which the observer dips into the stream and fills—not always to the brim—and which he then gazes at in undisturbed wonder. He gazes at the bowl and not at the river. The river cannot be dammed. It pays no heed to the attempts to dam it; it rushes on. The bowl, however, can be dipped into the stream and brought up at will.

It can be brought up and considered by itself. Once something is isolated from the flow of real objects—in our case the world—the question "What is it? What is it in essence?" is inevitably raised. And so once again the question is repeated. The answer to this question is always the same: Whatever it is, it is not what it appears to be.[32] And what does it appear to be? Well, the world. This, then, is mere appearance, an illusion [*Schein*]. But what is it in truth—"essentially"?

Several answers suggest themselves; and each of these answers represents the phenomenon seen from a certain point of view. First and foremost, it may be considered mere appearance, an illusion. Here we refrain from expressing its "essence" further, and catch hold of this single statement. Nevertheless we delve beneath the surface. A glance is sufficient to clear up the "mystery of essence" for us; we come to the conclusion that beneath the surface there is nothing. The essence of the world then is, Nothing.[33] A number of world views and even religions have happily attained to this ultimate wisdom.

It is also possible to begin with the assumption that appearance conceals "something" which is not mere appearance. The world, then, is not what it appears to be, but is something entirely different. It is unfortunate that so little is left in the world which can be entirely different. That all-inclusive term "world" includes so much. Two words, however, do escape by the skin of their teeth. The first of these words is "I," and there can be no doubt that it has had great popularity with the philosophers. After all, who is it that encounters the world? I do. Confronted by the world, my "ego" retained. I think, therefore I am. My "ego" is the only certainty. The world is appearance, illusion. However, it does appear to me; this is more than mere illusion. This is "essence," and it is concluded that the "ego" is the essence of the world. All the wisdom of philosophy can be summed up in this sentence. Of course there are distinctions and "schools of thought," and I am told that these distinctions are weighty and important.

And yet all the efforts, no matter how sublime or subtle, to bolster these distinctions are to no avail. There is no reason to assign to the "ego" a certainty which it cannot maintain. My own "ego" can certainly not lay claim to such a privileged position. Inasmuch as it is mine it is a part of the world and hence not distinguished from any other "ego" which it encounters. Any claim to the contrary must be based upon that which is suprapersonal in my "ego"—that is, its ability to become aware of its distinctive individuality. Strictly speaking, it is only my consciousness of self that I cannot encounter beyond the realm of myself. And yet, when taken as a dictum, such consciousness is encountered outside my self. I am forced to accept, for better or worse, the statement of others that they also possess consciousness of self, although in their case it is a consciousness of their selves not mine. It would seem to follow that the world possess as many "essences" as there are "egos" with separate consciousnesses. To avoid this absurd conclusion we are forced to revert to some abstract consciousness-in-itself. Of this "consciousness-in-itself," however, we know nothing. And furthermore the definition of pure suprapersonal consciousness excludes the possibility of knowledge. And so the "ego" is thwarted in its attempt to become the essence of the world; it turns out to be nothing. It is neither "subject" nor "object"—nothing. To justify its claims it must be nothing. The result: the essence of the world is "nothing"; nothing is at the core of the "world of appearance." It seems we have been overcharged for this delicious bit of information.

At this point we are informed that the fault rests with us. We have undertaken a fallacious enterprise—philosophy. This much philosophy understood correctly—the world must be something other than it appears to be. But this something cannot be identified with the Self. The "ego" also dwells in the world and is perhaps the most problematic of all "appearances." That which exists behind and beneath appearance, has to be something wholly other. The world appears to the Self, but conversely the Self also appears to the world. The witness is witnessed while witnessing. The astonishing fact about the world's appearance is not that there is someone to whom it appears. That a lucent eye catches sight of a sunbeam does not explain the luminary. It is the sunlight which illuminates the eye, dispels its darkness and acts upon the iris which mirrors its rays. The brilliance of light informs us of an illuminating source. No blaze without a fire. Light may shine without an eye to see, but not without a source. It is not man to whom light appears, but He who kindles the light, the illuminator, not the illuminated, who is concealed behind appearance. God, not man, exists behind the world.

God? Who is He? We have just detected the emptiness of the argument which posits the "ego" as world-essence. Is this another attempt to deceive us by a second empty word? We know that inevitably we will be given the answer of the mystics. But does mysticism make out a better case than philosophy? What can one comprehend of Him except that He is "wholly other" than the world and therefore its essence? Can one dare to call anything, anything at all, in this world of appearances, divine? This would be sufficient to divest God of His one significant function: to be wholly other than the world. The world, it was claimed, is appearance, and nothing but appearance: would any manifestation of God within the world then be a mere reflection of appearance? Everything in the world which bears the name of God—the burning faith deep in the heart of men as well as the flame dedicated to Him at the altar—must be considered merely shimmer and appearance. Such a God can have nothing in common with the God who acts as trustee of the world as it "appears," and of all "appearance." There is a remarkable resemblance between this God, the trustee of appearance, and the Self, in which appearance reappears. A God who deviates even by a hair's breadth from sheer, absolute nothing cannot be accepted as transcending appearance. To be essence He must be nothing. Again we have attempted to pierce the veil of appearance, and again all we have to show for our pains is nothing. Truly, once again, we have been overcharged.

Is *nothing* truly the "order" which is the essence behind appearance —pure, unadulterated appearance as well as the appearance of something, to somebody, about something? Is there no other way out? Is it not possible that appearance is everything and everything is only appearance? Is it not possible that there is nothing beyond appearance, not even something "wholly other"? And, if this is granted, can we not say that the world is everything [*Alles*]? Thus man, himself appearance, reflects a segment of the mirage, or, indeed, (why not?) the complete mirage. And God is merely the shadow cast by the frame of the mirror, or possibly the reflection of the mirror's glass.

This *is* undoubtedly the world with which we are so well acquainted. It is a world unaware of an Outside, of Before and After, of Hither and Yon, of Foremost and Hindmost, a world which refuses to acknowledge anything but itself. And even this acknowledgment is negated by its view that its very own self is mere appearance, illuminated by nothing and illuminating nothing. It is a world which has no reality beyond appearance, which is made up of multilateral refractions of appearance, appearance irradiated by appearance and the source itself of more appearance, reflecting nothing but appearance. There are no limits to this universal interaction of appearances. It is futile therefore to consider it as a whole; a whole would have boundaries and their shape would be a reality and not merely the reflection of an appearance.

Yes, indeed, we know this world. It belongs to "science" which at the present time constitutes a power next to "philosophy" and "mysticism." It presents unlimited claims and yet is easily satisfied. The discovery of a new beam of experience makes it happy; it would be contented if it could obtain another ray by rearrangement of the points of irradiation; such contentment is gained daily. The ultimate in satisfaction would be reached if science could chart the infinite possibilities of the reflections and deflections of appearance. This is a satisfaction that can never be had.

The essence of the world is appearance, boundless and undetermined. The undetermined character of appearance is thus, nothingness. It is nothingness which must be reaffirmed incessantly. In this respect it is unlike that nothingness which is commonly accepted as self-evident, by those who regard the world as sheer appearance from the very first. It is rather a nothingness which only becomes aware of its true character when it arrives at the conclusion that it will never reach its goal. It becomes aware of itself as nothingness if it does not deceive itself by the paradoxical concept of approximating the infinite—a paradox obvious to any student of mathematics, although it seems to frustrate our scholars. The sum of all appearances does not create Being; this could only happen if appearance ceased to be appearance. And that the world *is* appearance is the very foundation of this particular world-view. Being must be a stable something, not an appearance, in brief not an "essence"; it must *be*.

Is this perhaps the answer? All other answers to our question concerning the essence of the world of appearances have proved fruitless. We found that the answers, "Nothing," "I," "God," "Everything," were all reducible to the first answer, namely "Nothing." Does this last possible answer survive the test of such a reduction? Are we justified in saying that the world is—something?[34]

"Something" is a simple word. Is it too trivial in its simplicity? Can such a word serve as a proper answer? Is it not lightly used by exasperated parents to allay the curiosity of their children? And furthermore, even if we take this answer seriously, even if we say "the world is something," is this not an example of the "it is truly" type of answer, the acceptance of which cannot be expected from simple common sense? Yes, we have here an "it is" answer, but why? Since the question inquired about "essence," the answer that it elicited had to be in a corresponding form. Our answer is, however, characterized by a lack of presumption, quite unlike those answers which insisted on plumbing the "deeper regions" in order to demonstrate "essence." The latter pretended to ultimate profundity, while ours does not desire to be profound, but prefers to keep to the surface. It does not wish to speak of an ultimate issue but of primary ones. It does not wish a person to remain with it. It must be just a beginning. It does not claim to be truth —it does, however, aspire to *become* true. Thus it is merely a diving board.

To dive from this board is neither impossible nor difficult. A man destroys any possibility of acquiring knowledge of the world unless he begins with the commonplace that the world is something rather than nothing, something—not I, not God, not everything. It does not matter whether this course is taken consciously as a thinking person might take it, or unconsciously in the process of living. Man takes his first step towards an answer as part of the continuing process of life and of thought. Having served its initiation purpose, it turns out that there is nothing final about the answer, that it is as inadequate and incorrect as the question which brought it into existence.

The world is something. That is to say, it is not nothing; neither is it everything. There are other entities. This preliminary knowledge presupposes that the other entities, namely God and I, are at every moment accessible to the world, reach the world. Mention of the world requires the very next instant mention of man and God. The world is something only because it enters the stream to which it and everything else belongs. It is drawn into the stream by something which is not a part of the world, yet does not claim to be its "essence." The world clings to this something in a purely external manner, indicating thereby that there is something which may be considered outside of the world. God and man are truly external to the world, not its interior, nor "essence." By saying that the world is something, we merely express the fact that it is neither man nor God, that neither constitute its "essence." Thus at last we discover something which is the companion of everything, including every event which takes place in the world, and yet is external to them all: the Word. Language is not the world, nor does it make such claims. What actually is it? Unlike "thought," language cannot presume to be the "essence" of the world. If the world is something which permits the existence of other things exterior to the world but not its essence, there is only one thing that language can be; it must be a bridge between the world and these other things. And that is precisely what it is.

What spans the gap between my Self and the world? Moreover, since I am a part of the world, its citizen, how can I make a distinction between my Self and the world? Am I not merely a part among parts, a citizen among other citizens? The argument that I think the world, that I mirror it in thought and observation turns out to be invalid since the world, in return, mirrors my Self even as it thinks and observes. Therefore my thought cannot be the world's essence; and indeed the contrary assumption forced us to reduce thought to the nothing that it is. Language makes no such claims. It neither can, nor does it want to be, the world's essence. It only names the things of the world. Adam gives names; words find their way to things. To utter a word is to affix a seal as a witness of man's presence. The word is not part of the world; it is the seal of man.

Is it exclusively this? Then sick reason's characteristic distrust of words is justified. After all, at some point man must have *begun* to name. Even today it is frequently possible to determine when a thing was assigned a name, when it was discovered in its seclusion. In addition, human language is equivocal; a thing is besieged by a multitude of words, and scarcely two of them have precisely the same meaning. People speaking the same language may not even understand each other. What bearing, then, does the word have upon the thing to which it belongs? Obviously the words of humans are in themselves insufficient. In addition, there must be the certainty that what the individual has begun by his act of naming will be continued until the ultimate goal of common language is reached. Each word, as soon as it comes into existence, requires the strength of continuation and the capacity to traverse the river of time so that it may finally become the ultimate word. The word of man, an initial word whenever it is uttered by man, joins that which was ultimate from the first, the word of God. The intention of language to form composite designations and double names, its capacity to create such designations, is shown by the way things obtain a name whenever someone confronts them. To name is the primal right of all men, a right which they are forever exercising. The one condition required is that the creator of the name actually confront the thing. At this stage the name is only a cognomen. And then also the person, or persons, to whom the originator of the name exhibits the thing, must be present. Thus Adam performed the act of naming, and so also do his offspring.

In addition to these names, a thing has names which it does not receive. It already possesses them. They also may have been "cognomens," at some moment uttered for the first time. However, as soon as they are spoken, they adhere to the thing. From then on the thing goes by that name. The thing possesses equally the right to keep the name it has, and to receive new names. Whoever gave the old name may be absent or even dead; in spite of this the name he gave still clings to the thing. And furthermore each new name must come to terms with the old ones. The thing gathers names, and indeed its capacity to do this is inexhaustible. It is man's privilege to give new names. It is his duty to use the old ones, a duty which he must perform, though unwillingly. His obligation to pass on the old names, to appropriate them and translate them into names he himself designates—this creates the continuity of mankind. Mankind is always absent. Present is a man, this fellow or that one. The thing, however, is tied to all of mankind by language and by its inherent law of transmission and translation. These linguistic laws require that each new word confront the old.

And where does the presence of mankind manifest itself? Not in the word of man, of course, but in that of God. It is not entirely by accident that the Bible is the most widely translated of all books. (It is probably the first book of consequence to have been translated.) The word of God implies the certainty that it will become the word of all. We say there is a certainty, not merely a probability. There is no one for whom the word of God is not meant, whose presence is not implied by it; the word of man implies the presence of the speaker and someone to whom his speech is addressed—and so also with the word of God. If it were not necessary that the word of God become the word of all, we should consider the existence of such a possibility just one of the aspects of "civilization," or something of the sort. But it is not enough to rely upon the good intentions of man to integrate his own newly formed names into the context of all names which have been designated and are yet to be designated. Man is under the obligation to exact such an integration. He is in need of those names which are absent. He needs all of them without exception. Although they should remain forever absent, he must nevertheless take them into account. Being absent, they do not force themselves upon man's attention; but He, for whom both he and they are present, forces man to pay attention. And thus things insist on their privilege of being named and going by a name.

There is no thing which does not share in the language of man and God through its name, through the innumerable words spoken in its vicinity. Language stamps the sign of God and man upon all the things of this world. That a thing is considered something by the world gives it its continuity. The thing is not an appearance, an illusion; it is something. The thing does not gain in definition by being isolated and made stagnant; certainty of being "something" is not achieved by plumbing the depths of such an entity, but rather by opening the floodgates and permitting the stream of which it is part to inundate it. Our patient found himself incapable of purchasing a slab of butter because he could no longer avail himself of his God-given right, his privilege as a man, of conferring names. He had lost faith in the continuity of names and of other things; he had renounced his human privilege. And it was because he did not believe in the divine quality of language that he became uncertain of the names which he and others assigned to things. This necessarily followed from his insistence that the word "be" the thing, that his word be the word of others. We have learned that this is something that must be foregone. The thing is and as such immediately acquires a name. Its name bears it into the flow of things, and hence the question concerning the essence of things becomes meaningless. Even the world turns out to be only a segment of the whole, not an "essence," a part to which, like to other parts, something may occur [*geschehen*].

Three forces, thus, act upon even the smallest thing. Any thing is part of the world, and receives its name through man. God pronounces the judgment of fate upon this carrier of many names. New "things" are happening at every stage in this process, and they become events. This course of events, originating in things, never comes to an end. Since the world of things is itself only a segment of the whole, it suffers —as any something must, even as the whole does—the process of history and it is through this process that it is realized. The world is real only insofar as it enters into this process, a process which brings all of it within the context of the human word and God's sentence. The world as such does not exist. To speak of the world is to speak of a world which is ours and God's. It becomes the world as it becomes man's and God's world. Every word spoken within its confines furthers this end.

This is the ultimate secret of the world. Or rather, this would be its ultimate secret, if there were anything secret. But common sense blurts out this secret every day. As for common sense, it regards each day as final, "ultimate." We face the world each day innocently and fearlessly, considering it as the ultimate that it is; we confront all of its reality, willing to submit to each name. We are certain that our names are the names of things and that the name we bestow will be confirmed by God.

And thus each day we solve the ultimate question, frankly confronting each thing as we encounter it; we look for nothing beyond, do not try to walk suspiciously around the object; nor do we peer into its depths, but accept it rather as it is, as it hastens towards us. And then we leave it behind and wait for whatever is to come tomorrow.

CHAPTER **7** *The Cure: Second Week*

Life is not the most precious of all things; nevertheless it is beautiful. And what is life? This obviously is not the same question we asked last week—our question concerning the world. Man has a view of life—*Lebensanschauung*—and this is a different matter from having an opinion about the world—*Weltanschauung*. We do not acquire a view of life; we are born with it. At any rate one day we notice that we possess one. Somehow or other it is a part of being human. What is life? And what is man? These are one and the same question asked in different terms.

What is man?[35] What am I? Again the question is an ultimate one involving essence, a "what is it" question. This time, however, the inquiry is not about the "It" of the world but rather about the "ego" of man. Again an easy answer is on hand. Whatever this "ego" may be, it is certainly not what appears to me. It cannot be simply my "ego," that "ego" which constantly shows up in all experience and even beyond experience constantly ready to encounter life once more. This is certainly delusion, perhaps self-delusion. Though it confounds both deceiver and deceived, yet it remains deception.

But why must we accept this answer? Is it not because of the way the question has been posed? The nature of such an answer, beginning with "It is," requires that the predicate give additional knowledge. The predicate must add to our wisdom; it must have more of essence about it, be closer to the truth, if by only a hair, than the subject—as for instance four is as regards two times two. If I extract my "ego" from the environment in which it exists, if I observe it in isolation, then it immediately dissolves into hundreds of experiences scarcely distinguishable from each other. It will be difficult to discover a relationship between the "being" I was yesterday and the "being" I am today, or rather, with my present experience; equally difficult to discover will be the relationship between the "being" I will be tomorrow and tomorrow's experiences. The "ego" cannot be saved.

Is this actually so? A voice gives us contradictory advice; the "ego" must be saved. We must cling to it desperately, reflect on it, penetrate to its depths. Its surface, of course, is nothing but self-delusion but in its interior its essence will be revealed to us, that hiding place which the "ego" seeks and must then find. Beware of him who despairs and agrees to doubt with you. Beware of that straying mind whose "ego" has dissipated into thin air. Do not believe his loud assertion that the "ego" is nothing. The poor misguided fellow does not know that, if we are to enjoy life, we ourselves must give it significance. And even if he wishes to dispute that life has value, he first must live. Whether one doubts or believes, one cannot dispense with the "ego," with ourselves.

This indispensable Self is by no means identical with that Self which we found it impossible to save. Abandon that which is beyond recovery, let it fragment into its elements of personal experience, this is not that Self which is indispensable. To doubt or to believe, for yea or for nay, one requires that other Self which dwells beneath self-deception in the hidden house of essence. You lose your "ego" only insofar as you insist that it remain personal. Praise it; it lives beyond the narrow confines of your being in which it seemed to be imprisoned. Invest it with the authority for which it was ordained, and not only your own Self, but the whole world with its idols and gods, will be subject to you. There is nothing but you, if you will it so. If you liberate your will from petty stubbornness, it becomes omnipotent volition—God; within you, it is

God who wills; you are merely His tool, His voice. True, then, your Self is only a deception, a self-deception. But have the courage to be God. There is no God if you are willing to take upon yourself His office. Should you refuse to do this and deprive your Self of being God, how can such a Self endure God's existence?[36]

Madness! another voice shouts. What absurdity! First you believe that your Self, as a reflection of the "ego" within you, is self-delusion, and then you inflate the Self until it is too large to pass for deception; you regard it as not deception, if it is God's self-delusion. You are a fool and you know it, and that is all you know. Who, then, is the deceiver? An "ego" even the hugest "ego," would only deceive itself, if it believed that beyond its needs and desires, its knowledge and requirements, another "ego" was hidden which also needed and desired and knew.

The magician who dwells in the cave below the Self cannot be another "ego"; this which releases the effervescence of your petty self as well as the giant bubble of divine consciousness must be an altogether different entity. You dare not name that from which the divine and human "egos" emerge, which relinquishing them, allows them to brighten the short spans of their existence with dreams of power and feeling. You dare not name such an entity because you lack the courage to live without deceit. Your wretched little wisp of life must be in the center of the universe, and should you sneeze, you expect the stars to come tumbling down.

Pretending to the throne of the world, you are expelled from your own home; it is what you deserve; your pretentions made you despise your rightful place and you acted as though you headed a government of the world in exile instead of taking care of your house. The world can safely leave you to your pretensions; you are incapable of making a single move on its chessboard. And even were you to attain to the authority you claim, you would be incapable of doing more than confirm the statutes already in existence. Through the eyes of your giant, self-inflated ego, absolute nothing grins—absolute nothing which neither knows nor feels nor wants.

I fortunately have recognized my proper place from which nothing can budge me. The law of the world is my law; to obey it willingly, my duty and privilege. There is only one world and it is ruled by a single law. This world and this law determine even that ignorant self-delusion which believes itself independent of such law. Your Self is of the world, a part of it—nothing more. It has become detached according to the principles of eternal law, just as the bough sprouts from the tree, the sprig from the branch, and finally the leaves and blossoms from the sprig. Each believes itself to be more than it is; sprig believes itself to be branch, leaf, sprig, blossom, leaf—each a complete Self, and yet they are Selves only through that law which brings forth the sprout from the tree and permits it to feed upon it, age with it, die and disappear. The blossom may believe that its will determined the number of its leaves and the form of its seed, that it created the laws which ruled the tree— it may believe this, but soon it withers away and as it drops from the tree it wakes from its delusive dream. But the law of the tree remains unaltered. And so also the world remains unaltered while the dance of the Self, the witches' dance of human "egos" and deified "egos" continues, forever creating new steps and yet repeating the same pattern.

But let us pause a moment and have a closer look at this world which you have erected as a foundation underlying my "ego." You speak of its law in much the same way as your adversary spoke of the will of God. You attacked his position maintaining that whatever he said of God's will, I could say of mine as well. You argued that he could know nothing about God's will, since such a will could not properly serve as the essence of mine. God was allowed to will, think, know, only as I will and think and know. His own will, thought, and knowledge had to be completely vacant of personality, if my dream of being a self was not to be destroyed. It was necessary that his will be nothing, or else it became impossible for me to deceive myself into the belief that *I* was something.

In precisely the same way, you now empty your law of all the qualities one might expect a world law to have. The tree which you describe has no bark of its own, no roots. It consists entirely of sprigs and leaves and blossoms. Where then is the law of the tree appointing you to the post in which you have established yourself? Where is this secret word which does not care to divulge itself? You are not, as you wish us to believe, the bearer of the world's law. You have appointed your own kind as law of the world; all turns into a black nothingness unless you

78

color the world—yours are the tinges that illuminate it. Your antagonist received his authority from pale nothing, and you would like to derive your dignity from a nothing that is black. Unless you stand on your own, unless you live independently, neither God nor the world can help you. No matter whether you deceive in the guise of master or knave, whether you prefer to deceive by your deceit or be deceived by it, your acts and transactions are fraudulent. Be yourself. Be what you are, a human being, or else renounce yourself.

Very well then, let us adopt the other possibility. Let us not seek for anything beyond ourselves. Let us be ourselves and nothing more. Such a moment of existence may be nothing but delusion; we shall, however, choose to remain within the moment, deceived by it and deceiving it, rather than live in deception above or below the moment. Let our personal experience, even though it change from instant to instant, be reality. Let man become the bearer of these shifting images. It is preferable that he change masks a hundred times a day (at least they do belong to him) rather than wear continually the mask of the divine ruler of the world (gained by thievery) or that of the world's bond-servant (forced upon him). The hundred masks will serve in lieu of one countenance. Whenever I encounter man, I shall steep my countenance in his until it reflects his every feature. Even should I confront only the shadow of a face, buried deep in the mute and accusing eyes of an animal or in the silent gaze of ancient ritual stones, I shall submerge myself in them until I have absorbed their countenances and thus come in contact with everything that ever existed. Thus, traveling about the earth, I shall come face to face with my own Self. The innumerable masks of the innumerable instants, yours and mine, they are my countenance.

My face? Would I then find myself? Do I find myself, finding the world, deciphering everything that ever wore human features? The human eye may well have drunk in the dying murmurs of the sea and witnessed the waning stars of the nocturnal sky. Thus it is possible that I have participated in every spark of life, whether animal, man or God, which ever glowed within the expanse of sea or sky—but where has my own life gone, where shall it find a dwelling-place? What fate awaits the traveler who voyages to every shore? He is estranged from his own hearth, and yet he seeks his image there, unaware that his Self watches him through the ancient flames burning on the stationary hearth-stones. Did our traveler forget that he is only a shadow of himself, a nothing, deluding himself and others by the innumerable masks he wears? Indeed he has shared in all lives but his own.

So it turns out that no matter what we do the life of man dissolves into nothing. We heeded him who promised salvation by divinizing human life, and it was to no avail. His God we discovered was nothing. We went the way prescribed by him who said we should be saved if we submitted to the law of the world—but in vain. His world was also nothing. And finally we attempted to live life, without dependence, with complete self-reliance, all of life—and our own life becomes nothing. Nothing, always nothing. We seek a life which is something—not everything, only something, but a something which truly is.

Again we must deal carefully with that ever-recurring question, "What actually is it?"; again we must remember that when we reply to that question, "something," this is in reality not an answer but only a point of departure, a starting point. What is revealed is that he who seeks to find out everything through life and through life alone discovers nothing. Just as we caught hold of a world existing in the realm of God and man, we must daringly seize upon a life which is content to be an in-between state, merely a transition from one thing to another. Let us reject the ever-present answer, "Life is," "Man is—" and let us become part of the onward-moving life of man. Here life "is" not, it simply occurs [*geschieht*].

Once again it is language which erects the visible bridge from man to that which is not man, to the "other." A person's name, his first name, is so external [*äusserlich*] to him, that it is sufficient witness to the fact that there is something exterior to man, a "without" [*Aussen*] surrounding him. Man, however, attempts to invalidate this testimony by use of the little word "merely," merely a name. This "merely" implies that he might have a different name (how true this is). He received his name from his parents (what a profound observation!) and he could if he wished change it legally (an argument of incontrovertible validity). To sum up: a name is an intrinsically human affair; but this does not mean that it does not differ from other intrinsically human matters. The very acute observations which we have seen advanced as objections form the basis of this difference: a name is external to a person. When, then, is a name required, and what happens to a man when his name is spoken?

Here, again, the answer is simple. It can be seen most clearly in the case of a somnambulist or a person only half alive. He is forced into the presence of mind, to the internal, to himself. And where was he before? He dwelt in the past, in the "external," completely dominated by it. He was a particle in the world, ruled by its laws—laws which are always the laws of the past and which always act from without. His name liberated him from these laws. It recalls him from the world in which he was imprisoned, and returns him to his Self which, once his name is uttered, is free of the past, devoid of the external. Suddenly, hearing his name spoken, man knows that he is himself. He recognizes that he has the ability to begin again. But what, we wonder, enables him to be himself, to start all over? What gives him this spiritual power, this capacity to discover himself as present? His name represents permanence; it is the only tangible thing giving continuity to man's existence. Is it possible, then, that that which is permanent endows man with power over the moment?—for to discover oneself as present occurs in the instant. Is this the permanent essence of man—to be present to himself? Essence again? In spite of everything?

No, this is definitely not essence. How can a moment constitute "essence"—the moment which is forever disappearing, forever being devoured by the past? If the moment were essence, human freedom would suffer irreparable damage. It would be eternally swallowed up in the concatenation of cause and effect which is the law of the world. If freedom is to be the essence of man, it will pay dearly for such pretensions. The moment cannot be "essence." The moment cannot be at all. And even if it could exist, it is already gone, it has turned into the past. It cannot struggle, not even for an instant, against the pull of the past. And so the moment must be lost, and with it the present, and with it man's being present to himself.

To escape the power of the past, to transcend the law which constitutes causation, the moment must, at each instant, be reborn. This continuous renewal and resumption of the present is a contribution of the future. The future is the inexhaustible well from which moments are drawn; every instant new-born moments rise and replace the moments disappearing into the past. At each moment the future presents to man the gift of being present to himself. And so man may use his moments freely and then deposit them in the vast receptacle of the past. In the enduring process of receiving and using his moments he is man, master of the present, of his present—for it is truly his, if it is present. It is indeed born anew each instant, and each instant it dies.

Even his proper name bears witness that man has a twofold nature, that he is a child of the world and a child of God. Man has two names: a family name—or at least the name of his father—and a proper name. Through his surname, man belongs to the past; all that coerces him is contained in that name. Fate has a hold on him, and his surname is the gate by which fate enters—the gate cannot be entirely closed—enters and bears down on him. His other name is his proper name. His parents chose it, and in choosing it drew a line of demarcation beyond which fate cannot trespass. A man's proper name serves as a declaration that this is to be a new human being; it lays claim to the present by confronting man with a future. It always bears with it dreams and desires. And this is true, perhaps even more so, when a new-born child is "named" after someone. Such an act of naming expresses that the child be like "him" for whom he is named.

However, just as a surname does not compel a man to enter upon his inheritance, so giving him a proper name does not generate magical powers. His name neither coerces man nor gives him freedom; it merely indicates, it is only a sign post. And indeed it is a sign. His name refers man to something beyond himself; through it comes the compelling word of memory and the liberating word of hope. Because of it, he cannot even hope to remain in isolation. His double name reminds him that he can only be a child of man if he does not refuse to be a child of the world and God as well. These latter powers exert their reality by speaking through the mouth of his environment. Can they, addressing him by his family name, coerce him? No, he both wants and does not want to be coerced by them. The ever-passing world speaks through his mouth. And does the man who calls him by his proper name wish to free him? Scarcely ever; perhaps he even attempts to make his life conform to a certain attitude; and yet he does liberate him, though not intending to; he summons him to live his particular and unique present. The future, alive with dreams and desires, speaks through his mouth. Through the voice of many callers, a single voice calls. Each call summons to the future. Who is the caller?

This again is the ultimate secret, and again it is no secret at all. It was never hidden to the healthy. For have not men always understood when they were in full possession of their senses, when they did not fall prey to that madness which robs a man of his capacity to know himself and the present? Did they not always act in accordance with this secret when their trust in themselves was not undermined, and they refused to be enslaved by the laws of yesterday? Was this not no secret at all when they cast from themselves the burden and responsibilities of the ever-dissolving present and had access to that source which forever renews the present? And you, have you not always had the courage to live when you simply proceeded on your way, with the past at your heels, and the light of a dawning tomorrow already touching your brow?

CHAPTER **8** *The Cure: Third Week*

God—who is God?[37] It is beyond the capacity of man to fathom God, it is said. Even if this be true, we have discovered that the same can be said of man and the world. We could discover no answer, or at best fallacious answers, to our questions, What "is" man? What "is" the world? So we are scarcely surprised to hear this statement about God. Statements about the essence of God are given more timidly perhaps than about the essence of man and the world. And yet they are certainly given. They are given even more frequently. The philosophic coterie, and mankind in general, as soon as it begins to philosophize, has a special liking for them. In spite of the modern predeliction for *Weltanschauung* and *Lebensanschauung,* God still remains the favorite subject of philosophy. Metaphysics began as the science of God and it has never changed. If one investigates the views of the great philosophers, one makes the following odd discovery: none of them, up to Schopenhauer, would admit to being an atheist. Indeed, just shortly before Schopenhauer's time, one of the "greats" fought the view that his teachings were atheistic, as though his personal honor were at stake.[38] Schopenhauer, however, openly declared that he was not concerned with God. He made atheism respectable. Even if this were his only merit, he would deserve to be commended.

This is, as a matter of fact, one of the answers that can be given concerning the essence of God. As in the case of man and the world, this question again presupposes that whatever knowledge we have is held precariously. Our knowledge of our various "gods and idols" seems at first to consist of nothing but fanciful imagery. But, it is maintained, these creations of ours may stand for something real. On the other hand, they may have no foundation in reality whatsoever. They may have been created by fear, lust, a creative instinct, a desire to explain, etc. It is necessary to entertain openly that they are possibly nothing, unreal. Moreover, the man who takes such a point of view should not be accused of ignorance nor threatened with ignominy. As posed, the question requires this answer, among other answers, as does every question which asks about the essence of a particular phenomenon or appearance.

Anyone who seeks another answer finds once again that he is faced with two alternatives. Both of these alternatives rest on the assumption that "something" exists behind appearance which is "altogether different" from what appears. They either assume that there is a fantast concealed behind our phantasmagoria who indulges in fantasies "within ourselves," very much like raving children in certain types of delirium appear to be possessed by an alter-ego which seems to be their nature and yet is not their true self. Or they conceive of a phantom-reality existing behind the images we see, in much the same way as a frightened child transforms a white sheet into a ghost, or the design on the wallpaper into a gorgon's head. Mother's common sense will not hesitate to disabuse the child. The resourceful woman will not tell him that this delirious second self, these ghosts and contorted faces, are real. She will attempt to awaken the child, will teach him to distinguish the sheet and the wall-paper design from ghosts and apparitions, his self from that which is alien. Philosophy, however, takes a different attitude and finds itself in an alliance with sick reason; for either it attempts to construct a god from the alter ego which possesses the patient, or else from those objects which turned into phantoms.

Nature is God. So enthusiastic adolescents, snobbish striplings, and unthinking adults, from university lecturers on, repeat the message of the Dutch Jew.[39] These phantoms within us which we associate with God are explained by the white sheet that produced them. But the sheet is not the sheet, and God forbid that the world should be the world. The sheet and the ghost are "essentially" one; the world is God (in essence). Mother, having embroidered and hemmed the sheet, is quite well aware of the fact that her sheet is really a sheet. One would think that mankind, busily developing the technical possibilities of nature, would know better than to doubt that its world is *the world*. But no! it must be "God"—God, of all things. Such prattlers pretend to believe in nature and do not have the faintest notion of the injustice they do to it by depriving it of its reality and labelling it a phantom. What sort of faith is it which must rename the object of faith so it may believe in it? Ordinarily, to have something means to accept it just as it is. This is the way I have faith in an act of friendship or an item of information. If I seek for the "true attitude" behind the friendly act, for the "true facts" upon which the item is based, I merely demonstrate that I lack faith in them. This is, however, how these people believe in the world. They believe in it—or rather pretend to believe in it—only if they are permitted to give it another name—the name of God.

To be God, the world must be shelled and husked, deprived of its reality. Heaven forbid that the world should be an ordinary, natural world. It has to be viewed in ecstasy. Mother must not say that the sheet was bought and hemmed by herself, that it is merely a piece of linen, because in this way she would deprive her child of its nightmare. Baruch Spinoza was no Spinozist. The spirit of Spinoza's concept of nature was rarefied by Goethe and Herder. It was this deified "nature" robbed of all natural qualities, not Spinoza's *deus sive natura* which became the God of the enthusiasts. Only a voided and annihilated world, a world turned into nothing was approved of as the nature of God. The statement "God is the world" can be made only if the world is nothing.

I hear a voice cheering. "Go ahead," the voice says, "give a good beating to those who would transform God into nature and make Him all-embracing matter. However, you must exempt from your attacks that god who is Mind." My reply is that I shall never say anything against Him which has not already been said by those who profess faith in this God with every word they utter. The beginning of all their wisdom is that to fear God is an insane fancy. To discover the truth, they say, we need not consider him whom these phantoms signify, that is the feared Lord. Oh no! He is utterly inaccessible, completely unknowable, like all which is "deep" under the "surface." We need not even consider the occasion which induces the phantasm. We must consider, however, the fantast, that is, man in fear of God. Man and man's prostrate mind is to be the essence of God. Thus the mind of man has won a promotion. It is unfortunate but inevitable that it should lose the very quality which earned it its promotion, that is, that quality which permitted it to comprehend its limitations, namely, the fear of something higher than man. In its exalted condition it has no use for such a quality. It is impossible to assert, God is venerating mind. We must keep to the statement, God is Mind.

Consequently, mind, the human mind, becomes God's essence. And so man's fantasies of gods and spirits become fantasies of the one and only mind, which is now divine. We have already pointed out that elevating the human mind to the position of being God's essence deprived it of its intrinsic relationship to God, a relationship present in man's fantasies; in these fantasies God was feared and venerated, and also present in these fantasies was the longing for love and creativity and the thirst for knowledge. Now it becomes clear that man is perfectly capable of referring these feelings and qualities to himself. Man's mind is capable of loving, creating, and exploring itself. This is made possible by the fact that generation follows upon generation; the inherent possibilities of this situation are summed up in the words "development," "evolution." Thus to say that there is divine mind means that God Himself is mind, evolving and unfolding.[40] And consequently it is through evolution that the human mind's claim to be God's essence is validated. But what follows from this?

It follows from this that God is not. What does evolution or development mean when we speak of the human mind? When do I make much of the fact that I am still developing? Is it not when I am apologizing for a shortcoming, for not having accomplished something which was expected of me? Mind which requires further evolution is simply not yet Mind. A citizen of the future may be a wonderful person, but he

88

is nevertheless not a citizen of the present. A man who adores the world of his children may be esteemed by all, but he is no lover of his own world. A jack-of-all-trades is a dabbler in his own profession.

Man is privileged to have everything that he needs to be man. He is in possession of the moment. And as for the rest, God and the world assist him here. He is in possession of the moment and so he has everything. Thus he is enabled to fulfill the commandment given to him because the command is for the moment and always only for the moment. The person which he confronts represents the whole world and the very next instant may represent eternity.[41] But the notion of development deprives him of the privilege of being human—a privilege which is also a duty. Evolution takes the place of man. That human mind, which was proclaimed to be the essence of God, is consequently not the true mind. It is rather a mind deprived of its human privileges, a mind annihilated. Nothingness replaces the living human being and this nothingness is proclaimed to be the essence of God.

All that remains, then, is as we have seen twice before, the attempt to take this phantasm seriously. Let us seek for the essence in the heart of appearance not somewhere behind it; let us look for it not in a single phenomenon but in the abundant whole. God is thus not something wholly other, essentially mind or world, but everything. He is everything which at any time bore the name of God; all the gods and idols of man assemble and in their transient manifestations and transformations make up that which we call God. God is the sum of all of His manifestations, transient though they be. That is all. But if these manifestations are truly "everything," then all things, both human and of the world, must be contained in them. Each and everyone of the gods is a giant grave containing in it all of the men who professed faith in this god as well as the world in which their creativity enclosed him. Are these sepulchral vaults anything but giant, empty halls, graves of graves? Forgotten are the dead, covered by their tombstones; nothing remains but the stones, and these empty sepulchres of the departed gods —or rather of the god who dies in all gods. May he rest in peace!

We do not wish to disturb his slumber, and if we did we would find no corpses. All we would find is nothingness. If God is to be *something,* he can be neither mind nor nature; nor can he be everything. All such attempts lead to nothing. To be something he must be Something. World must be a Something, man a Something, God a Something.

Our reluctance to accept the notion of God being "Something" is incomparably stronger than our previous tendency to reject the idea of man and the world as "Something." In the latter case it was merely the trivial manner of expression which repelled us; but a touch of impropriety—indeed a suggestion of blasphemy—is added when we speak so of God. God—"Something"? Do others exist besides him? So the philosopher, and the man infected by philosophy (and after all who is not?) will express his doubts. And he will come to the conclusion that such a degradation of God must inevitably revolt the *homo religiosus,* a species which is a favorite topic with our philosopher; he certainly knows everything worth knowing. But his conclusion in this instance is by no means correct. Common sense knows as a matter of course—and common sense may even be encountered in this territory, covered though it is with philosophic mouse-traps—that I and God are not identical, nor is He identical with the tree I see in blossom before me, nor for that matter with any "ideal" ego I may possess, or any "final" ego I may aspire to. Common sense, on the contrary, will tend to think of such a confusion of God with other things and ideas as "pagan," and will attack it accordingly. However, how can common sense reconcile the two statements that God is "Something" and that man and the world are also "Something," inasmuch as it must admit that "to be Something" has a different meaning when it refers to God?

Of course, it does admit such a difference. This admission, however, grants merely—as in the case of man and the world—that the word "something" cannot adequately describe an essence. Common sense neither describes nor designates this essence; it makes no attempt to grasp it; no sooner has the thought "God is Something" occurred to common sense than the thought is left behind. Common sense expresses this thought and, as it does so, learns that God cannot be spoken of unless, at the very same moment, a bridge is constructed to man and the world.

What forces us, when we speak of God, to build such bridges? What quality of God is beyond the reach of all our ideas and fantasies? How does it happen that so many of our ideas of Him, in fact all of them, agree that he is One, unite in Him as One. What is there sufficiently external to God, yet despite its externality so inseparable from Him that it belongs to Him—what is there sufficiently "extrinsic" to reach across to that which is without?

It is His name. To utter God's name is entirely different from uttering the name of a man or a thing. True, they have something in common; the name of God, His proper name, and a term of designation are not identical with the bearers of these names. But except for this they differ widely. Man has a name so that he may be called by it. To be called by his name is for him an ultimate distinction. God does not have a name so that he may be called by it. To Him it is irrelevant whether His name is called or not; he heeds him who calls Him by His name as well as those who call Him by other names or those who speak to him in name-less silence. He bears a name for our sake, so that we may call Him. It is for our sake that He permits Himself to be named and called by that name, since it is only by jointly calling upon Him that we become a "We."

And thus the name of man remains a proper name and clings to him; He keeps the name bestowed on Him. God's name, however, is subject to change although, at any particular instant, it is conceived of as a proper name. Indeed the encounter with God is established and transmitted from place to place, from thing to thing, from man to man, from people to people, from order to order, by this very alteration of names.

In this respect the name of God resembles that of a thing. A noun does not remain at the place where it was first spoken. It may have originated as a proper name; when it becomes a noun not only does it reach many people—that happens to a proper name as well—but it also reaches many things. At this point a noun grows in size and intertwines with other words; thus words lose their meaning as .proper names, meanings which made them adhere, as it were, to individual things. Thus words intertwine and the unity of language is established. Here is a world in which many things are merged and resolved. The language of the individual, so far merely a personal world, begins to blend into the language of a people, and in turn the language of a people blands into that of mankind. And things are drawn along in the wake of this movement, proceeding from the single object designated in the Here and Now toward a more highly integrated world-order, toward the ultimate order.

The name of God proceeds on its way above these two movements, the movement of proper names towards the ultimate community and the movement of words denoting things towards the ultimate order—it proceeds on its way both as a name and as a term of designation, and it participates in both of the movements. Invoked by men as a name, it spreads itself above the congregations of men, the congregations with their originally divergent names; as a noun it consecrates things, and things are dedicated to it; thus it acts as a force gathering things and giving them order.

This dual task undertaken by the name of God—dual since in one aspect it concerns man, and in the other the world is reflected in its tendency to split and become a two-fold name.[42] Man invokes God by His name; the world speaks to Him through His word. On the one hand He embraces sinners; on the other, He proclaims law for the world. The root of all of man's various heresies is to confound the two parts of His name with one another; God's love encroaches upon His justice, His justice upon His love. It is indeed God's task both to maintain the two-fold character of His name as well as reconcile them. So long as there is reason for such a division, so long as God is not the God-in-Himself [Gott an sich] whom philosophers drivel about; if He remains God of man and the world, then it is He, who by means of His two-fold name transforms—and we use the word in its technical sense—human energies into the energies of the world.

Man and the world go their separate ways; and this cannot be, nor should it be, changed. Man should remain human; he should not be converted into a thing, a part of the world, prey to its organization. And the world's law and order should be neither rescinded nor sentimentalized. Man ought to be able to abide by the world's constitution, judge by its laws, measure according to its standards, and yet remain human. He should feel no necessity to withdraw from the world's order because of his humanity. He should not despair and leave unfilled his obligation to judge, to designate, to name those things which the world parades before him. Yet how could he act, were he not sure that his actions and the world-process, his sentiments and its order, interrelate and agree?

92

This certainty belongs to him and he is justified in keeping it. There is in addition to the world and himself, He who turns His face towards both. He it is who summons man by name and bids him take his place in the congregation who calls upon Him. He it is who orders things so that they may form a kingdom bearing His name. Thus man may act unconcerned with the outcome; he may act according to the requirements of the world as it is today. That day, the day when action is required, lets him understand what he must perform. The realm of time is the proper arena for his action. He does not need to wait until truth has risen from the depths. Truth waits for him; it stands before his eyes, it is "in thy heart and in thy mouth," within grasping distance; "that thou mayst do it."[43] In the same way as he has achieved certainty concerning the reality of the world and has found the courage to live his life, he must also have faith in Him who brought him into existance. It is at this very point that Hamlet, finding himself in the world, gives way to shame and despair. But even Hamlet persists in his despair only as long as he remains in soliloquy. As soon as the requirements of the moment take hold of him, once the solitude of his soliloquy is destroyed, he does the correct thing unhesitatingly and makes his disjointed world whole. When man is in need he depends on common sense; he has no time to waste on such a luxury as sick reason. The proper time then is the present—today. To avail himself of today, man must, for better or worse, put his trust in God.

Is this not the way things are with you? When need forces you into the present, do you still insist on asking about yesterday and tomorrow? Do you still require eternity to give you proof of the Here and Now? No, there is no time for such things. For the proper time has come, and thus God assists you.

CHAPTER **9** *Convalescence*

These have been strenuous weeks. The treatment was so intense the patient scarcely found time to rest. Therefore we cannot take the responsibility of returning him to his daily duties until he has received some urgently needed post-therapeutic treatment. We must see to it that he is placed in situations where the obstacles which he has learned to surmount are not erected artificially for training purposes but are arranged in a perfectly natural order. We believe that the past weeks of training have taught him not to shirk from obstacles, to handle them efficiently. It will however, be best to convert the skill he has acquired on the drill-grounds into habitual performance. A sudden shift to every day life, and perhaps an area entirely without obstacles, may result in a loss of the talents which he has acquired.

Where in every day life do we find areas in which God, world, and man are dealt with directly? Let us recall the trivial examples which we used at the outset to define the realm of common sense. We did not mention God, man or the world explicitly; we were concerned with a juridical decree, a proposal of marriage and a slab of butter. That is, we were concerned merely with parts, with fragmentary actions, and

95

not with the whole. With our training exercises it was otherwise; there we dealt with the whole. Our exercises, however, were so managed that in learning to deal with the whole, we also learned how to deal with the parts. But, at this point, we require some sphere of real life which has not been isolated for therapeutic purposes; a sphere if possible relating to the whole. Work days do not constitute such a segment.

Work days do not, but holidays do.[44] Although the holiday is also separated from the work day, the separation is natural. Although it is exceptional, it is an exception that appears regularly; it is the exception that proves the rule. It is through the holiday that the work day receives its definition. We must bear in mind that we are not dealing with something entirely distinct from the weekday world as though the serious side of life were now replaced by the elation of art. In such a case the exceptional is indeed exceptional and does not prove the rule. According to Schiller's[45] definition, which expresses the hitherto prevalent aesthetic attitude of classicism-romanticism, art is not life. It is not even a part of life, but belongs to an altogether different world, a world which finds its meaning and justification in its very otherness. Even its ultimate seriousness is a game; it plays its games seriously.

This is not the difference between holiday and work day. Insofar as the holiday is exceptional, it merely confirms the work day. There is no superior content to the holiday. The holiday does not seek that which is absent from the work day, does not know what the work day is not capable of recognizing. It does, however, state explicitly and as a whole those things which the latter expresses only partially and occasionally. God, man, and the world are the content of the holiday, and in a perfectly everyday manner.

The holiday knows as little as the sane, healthy work day, what God, man, and the world "are." The holiday does not permit their "essences" to be disputed. It knows no remote God, no isolated man, no fenced-in world. God, man, and the world are for it in constant motion; they are in transition, the three of them constantly joining and interweaving and separating. The undulations of beseeching and receiving, receiving and thanking, go on incessantly. Man asks, God gives, the world receives and thanks—and then man asks anew. There can be no dead season, no merely localized pulsation here; the process must be continual. The holiday cannot pretend to isolate any of the three elements. It must do without the spectacle of drama, because unfortunately drama remains mere spectacle. A holiday must not isolate itself; a spectacle does precisely that. So does a holiday if it manifests itself as carnival or pageantry, or art-festival. The holiday which confirms the work day, which does not contradict it, is not closed off; it flows into other holidays. This chain of feast-days forms the festive year. At the end of the year this circle is closed. But here too there is no halt; there is rather a forward motion, a flowing on. Here too the holiday is like the work day—a progress, a transition, never a standstill. There is one difference, however; with the holidays a shape is achieved, a well-rounded form.

It may seem paradoxical at first that the occurrences of a holiday should be identical with those of the work day. They present such a dissimilar picture. What happens on the average week day? What rhythm dominates everyday occurrences? What pulsation appears in even the minutest phase? Throughout the day in every single breath inhalation gives way to exhalation; work is replaced by rest. And it is this which finally divides the day into its component halves of sleeping and waking.

In his waking state man is, as it were, at home with himself, a man among men, man confronting the world. If human life consisted only of the waking hours, man would be omnipotent, the world would be clay for his creative and creating hands, and man himself his own center, his own god. But such is not the case. Life does not consist only of the waking hours. Night begins; man rests. The world slips through his fingers, lies down at his side, surrounds and absorbs him. He ceases to be the center of things. He ceases to be, but the world *is*.

If the world were forever, if it alone existed, man would become merely one of its dreams, and the world would exist for itself entirely, and be its own god. But this too is not the case. Once more the day dawns, and man rises and begins the day's work. Neither man nor world exist by themselves. Neither *is*. If either *were* it would exist alone; the stream would cease to flow. It is the connective "and" that links day and night, that links waking and sleeping, that makes man and the world into a Something. This "and" is the work of Him who maintains the continuity of day and night, who gives the power of speech to day, and grants to nights its silence. By itself this connective could not exist.

But the three woven together form evening and morning into a day.[46]

Here, then, is the day, today and everyday, anyone's day, the work day. And here too is the holiday, for it is introduced in exactly the same way. It also contains two complementary occurrences, namely asking[47] and thanking. Who is the one who must ask? It is man, for he alone is capable of asking. Man asks—and it is for this reason that he was granted the gift of language. It is for this reason that his lips have been unsealed. And his requests cannot be gainsaid. Could he be forever asking, there would be no resisting him. A man who asks cannot be disregarded; one must turn away one's eyes to reject his entreaties. As long as one meets him face-to-face, his request must be granted. As long as man is face-to-face with other men, he is protected from violence, if he does not lose his courage and with it the power to ask.

To ask, to pray, is the most human of acts. Even man's silence may entreat; and mute nature acquires speech when it supplicates—as in the case of the silent eyes of an animal. Prayer awakens the man in man. A child demands with his first word. And the first word from him who awakens from the slumber of childhood is also a request, a prayer.

Yet man is not always capable of speech; he cannot always ask. He must be allowed to maintain his silence. In his prayers he is alone, a solitary human. "Help me, O Lord, for the waters have risen to my throat."[48] "My God, my God, why hast Thou forsaken me?"[49] But as he offers thanks, he goes forward to the whole world. The world must acquire the power of speech to include him. "Let everything that breathes, praise the Lord."[50] "To Thee silence is praise."[51] The silent world praises and thanks God; man mingles his praises with its. As he gives thanks he becomes part of the world. But if man only thanked, he would be swallowed up by the world; he would cease to be man. His voice would be barely audible in the chorus of praise sung by the world. But man is not swallowed up; he is confronted by his need again and again. He no sooner offers thanks than he must pray again for that which he requires next—his thanks are universal in intent, his prayer remains for the particular. Thus the cycle of events continues; and connecting prayer and thanksgiving, man and world, is He to whom they are addressed.

This is the way of holidays; they proceed unimpeded by the slow

Convalescence poetry of prayer or the more expansive strophes of thanksgiving. The holiday moves steadily from one to the other, and then back again—it is in continuous transition. This movement is identical with that which governs the work day. Here we discovered that waking and sleeping, tension and relaxation alternate; but generally the movement of the work day goes on in silence. In the holiday it finds vocal expression. Whoever has recognized the rhythmic movement of the latter, will not fail to yield to the rhythm of the former. The holiday will serve as a training school for every day. Once a man's legs are accustomed to its rhythms, he will have no difficulty walking the streets of the work-a-day world. The gait is the same. If he has been well-trained here, he will not stumble later. Rather he will halt in amazement at how simple life actually is.

CHAPTER **10** *Back to Work*

But is it entirely true that life is simple? Why does it seem more diffi-cult than we had expected? Have we not responded to the treatments, convalesced, and regained our common sense? Nevertheless we discover upon our return to everyday life that existence is still difficult. To have prayed and given thanksgiving on holidays is not enough. Life itself in-sists that it be lived. What are the consequences of this?

Did we not learn that we must not permit ourselves to be diverted and brought to a standstill, that we must never diverge from the way? We must never forget this lesson. But is this all that life requires? Is there not more?

No, this is all, but to accomplish this is difficult enough. Strength, a great deal of strength, is required since the stream of life flows uninter-ruptedly from its sources towards the estuary. The stream will never flow in the opposite direction. Life is not eternal life; it flows from birth towards death.[52] The days succeed each other in monotonous progres-sion. Only the holidays merge to form the yearly cycle. Only through the feast days is the everlastingness of the stream experienced; here one sees the stream forever returning on itself. Only here does life become eternal. Then weariness, and anxiety, and disappointment depart; the course of the river has been mapped, the river whose end and beginning are one. But weakness, anxiety, and disappointment exist on the work days; though life gains new strength from the holidays, it does so only to gain further frailties, anxieties and disappointments. The road stretches out before us, but it does not lead, as on feast days, to an ever-young eternity; it is an endless road, an infinite one, extending towards its ultimate end. Life moves towards death.

We have wrestled with the fear to live, with the desire to step outside of the current; now we may discover that reason's illness was merely an attempt to elude death. Man, chilled in the full current of life, sees, like that famous Indian prince, death waiting for him. So he steps outside of life. If living means dying, he prefers not to live. He chooses death in life. He escapes from the inevitability of death into the paralysis of artificial death. We have released him from his paralysis, but we are unable to prevent his death; no physician can do that. By teaching him to live again, we have taught him to move towards death; we have taught him to live, though each step he takes brings him closer to death.

Each step that he takes is accompanied by fear. This is not as it should be; the courage to face life should still all fear. Moreover this fear is not a fear of life; that fear has been overcome. It is no longer fear of the next step to be taken; the step has been taken, but once taken it becomes the cause of fear. Now that life is being lived, it is dreaded because it belongs to death. Fear turns to disappointment.

This also is not as it should be; such disappointments should not exist. Faith in God should never allow such disappointment to arise. What do I care about success? But disappointment is not really a doubt of success. Doubt can no longer plague me; my disappointment is rather concerning events that have passed. They should have been life itself—and yet they are already dead. It does not matter that they will generate life. Disappointment turns into weariness.

This, too, is not as it should be. The world's assurances should prevent one's eyes from closing. Nor do they close. They peer ahead to find what the hands must grip next and where the feet must step. They are not weary of life. Life continues, but they fear to look backwards, for there death is at work.

Back to Work   It is so difficult to realize that all verification lies ahead, that death is the ultimate verification of life, that to live means to die. He who withdraws from life may think that he has avoided death; however, he has merely foregone life, and death, instead of being avoided, closes in from all sides and creeps into one's very heart, a petrified heart. If he is to be restored to life he must recognize the sovereignty of death.

He must direct his life to no other goal but death. Only then does life become simple, inasmuch as it no longer seeks to elude death, being willing to chant the dirge at any moment, while advancing in the face of death. He must know that at the end of the path of graves, a grave is already being prepared for him.

There is no remedy for death; not even health. A healthy man, however, has the strength to continue towards the grave. The sick man invokes death and lets himself be carried away in mortal fear. In health, even death comes at the "proper" time. Health is on good terms with Death. It knows that when the Grim Reaper comes he will remove his stone mask and catch the flickering torch from the anxious and weary and disappointed hands of Brother Life; it knows that he will dash it on the ground and extinguish it, but it also knows that only then the full brilliance of the nocturnal sky will brightly glow. It knows that it will be accepted into the open arms of Death. Life's eloquent lips are put to silence and the eternally Taciturn One will speak: "Do you finally recognize me? I am your brother."

Epilogue to the "Expert"

Are you still around? Didn't you hear me? I had really hoped that you would have understood at least enough to prompt you to withdraw.

What did you say? Do I understand you correctly? Are you complaining? You have been bored? Did you say that we were wrong, that all this has already been said by Bergson?[53] We have added nothing new to your knowledge? Sir, do you presume that I am here to please you? You have no right to complain. If you have been bored you cannot hold me responsible. I stated explicitly that you would depart unrewarded. You should have taken my advice at face value. I definitely decline any responsibility. You have been warned in advance.

Epilogue to the Reader

You must be a little frightened. Contrary to our initial agreement we have dealt with serious matters. Certainly they have become more serious than you expected. The responsibility for that, however, does not rest with me. Life is a serious matter. Ordinarily you are aware of that yourself. You would strongly resent it if your work, your actions and your tribulations were not taken seriously. The things we dealt with are of the same order of seriousness. They are not more serious. But they are serious.

At this point we must part company. I hope that I am not bidding you farewell forever. We have had such a close acquaintanceship that I believe that many things remain to be said. Whenever you are able to spare some time come and visit me at my home. You will be welcome.

NOTES

1 Franz Rosenzweig, *Briefe,* ed. Edith Rosenzweig and Ernst Simon,
   Berlin 1935, p. 371.

2 *Franz Rosenzweig: His Life and Thought,* ed. N. N. Glatzer, New
   York 1953, pp. 94-98.

3 In 1925, Rosenzweig wrote "The New Thinking," a popular presentation of the background of *The Star of Redemption;* in this essay
   reappear a number of motives used in the present treatise.

4 Cf. on this subject: Sydney C. Rome, "Scottish Refutation of Berkeley's Immaterialism," *Philosophy and Phenomenological Research,*
   III (1943), 3.

5 *Briefe,* p. 406.

6 Hans Vaihinger, *Philosophie des Als-Ob,* 1911, pp. 684 f.

7 See H. Scholz, *Die Religionsphilosophie des Als-Ob,* Leipzig 1921.

8 *Ibid.,* XIV.

109

9 See W. M. Urban, *Language and Reality*, London 1939, pp. 52–56.

10 *Ibid.*, ch. VII and Appendix III.

11 *Nietzsches Werke*, VI, 43.

12 *Franz Rosenzweig: His Life and Thought*, pp. 198 ff.

13 *Briefe*, p. 407.

14 *Franz Rosenzweig: His Life and Thought*, pp. 144 f.

15 See Aphorism 78 in Franz Kafka, *The Great Wall of China*, New York 1946, p. 297.

16 Franz Kafka, *Hochzeitsvorbereitungen auf dem Lande*, New York 1953, p. 101.

17 *Franz Rosenzweig: His Life and Thought*, p. 160.

18 Franz Rosenzweig, *Kleinere Schriften*, Berlin 1937, p. 397.

19 *Franz Rosenzweig: His Life and Thought*, p. 286.

20 William James, *Pragmatism*, London 1907, p. 201. On Wm. James and Rosenzweig, see Ernst Simon in *Molad*, 1953, pp. 299–311.

21 Letter of December 24, 1922, to Martin Buber. *Briefe*, p. 469.

22 This refers to *The Star of Redemption* to which the writings that followed including the present treatise are here considered as prolegomena, or introductions.

23 The German word for "to wonder," marvel *[staunen]* means also to stand still. Cf. the obsolete "astound," which means both to strike with amazement and to stun, to stupefy.

24 The Latin *substantia is* derived from *sub*, under and *stare*, to stand: that which underlies all outward appearances. To Spinoza it means the eternal reality lying beneath the modes, individual forms and particular events; substance (which goes back to *ousia*, being of the Scholastics) is the "essence" of the world.

25 What follows are satirizing references to the "as if" philosophy of Hans Vaihinger. See Introduction.

26 This is an allusion to the initial lines of Goethe's *Faust*.

27 *Philosophie des Als-Ob*, which appeared in 1911, was written in 1876–78.

28 Rosenzweig dealt with the problem of "name" in *The Star of Redemption*, second part, second book; in some notes to *Judah ha-Levi* (see *Franz Rosenzweig: His Life and Thought*, p. 281) ; in the essay, "Der Ewige," in *Kleinere Schriften*, pp. 182–198.

Notes **29** This is an allusion to the activity of representatives of the Kantian Critique of Reason from Erhard Schmid and Karl Leonhard Reinhold, who introduced Kantian philosophy in the University of Jena, up to Vaihinger. Rosenzweig is opposed both to Kant's theory of knowledge and to any mystical avoidance of reality ("Mysticol injections").

30 A reference to world-man-God.

31 The contents of this chapter dealing with the view of the world corresponds to the second book of the first part of *The Star of Redemption*.

32 Considerable attention has been given to the problem of "appearance" also in philosophical literature in the English language, e.g., in *Appearance and Reality*, by Francis H. Bradley, London and New York 1893. — Rosenzweig's argument plays on the not merely linguistic relationship between the German *Erscheinung* (appearance) and *Schein* (illusion).

33 Cf. the statement by Friedrich Heinrich Jacobi, one of the first opponents of Kant: "In a twofold enchanter's smoke, called time and space, rise the ghostly forms of phenomena or appearances in which nothing appears." According to Jacobi, Kant's critical reason is busy about pure nothing, i.e., only about itself. Hegel gave up the idea that the world can be derived from the "nothing" of absolute indifference; he attempted to raise this empty substance to "mind": "the self-determined subject."

34 Rosenzweig's criticism of German idealism is presaged in the philosophy of Schelling in his last period. Schelling agreed with Hegel that logic in the metaphysical sense is at the basis of philosophical thought, but opposed the notion that logic is more than the negative aspect of existence. Logic or "pure thought" cannot explain existence, as Hegel had attempted. Schelling said: "The whole world lies, as it were, in the nets of understanding or of reason, but the question is *how* it came into these nets, since something else and something *more* than mere reason, indeed, even something striving beyond these limits, is evidently in the world" (*Sämmtliche Werke*, Stuttgart and Augsburg, 1856-61, First Division, vol. X, 143).

35 This chapter offering a view of man is paralleled by the third book of the first part of *The Star of Redemption*.

36 "If there were Gods, how could I bear to be no God? Consequently there are no Gods" (Nietzsche).

37 "God and his Being, or, Metaphysics" is the title of the first book of the first part of *The Star of Redemption*.

38 In 1799, Johann Gottlieb Fichte, Kant's greatest disciple, published a treatise, "On the Ground of our Belief in a Divine Governance of the World," which affirmed such a belief but rejected the existence of God "as a separate being." That gave rise to a fateful atheism-controversy. The Government of Saxony confiscated the treatise as "atheist."

39 Spinoza: "I say, All is in God; all lives and moves in God" (Letter 21, to Oldenburg). "By the help of God I mean the fixed and unchangeable order of nature, or the chain of natural events" (*Treatise on Religion and the State*, ch. 3). Ludwig Feuerbach: "Where God is being identified — or confounded — with nature or nature with God, there is neither God nor nature but a mystical amphibolic hybrid" (S. Rawidowicz, *Ludwig Feuerbachs Philosophie*, Berlin 1931, p. 181).

40 This refers to the Hegelian idea of the dialectically necessary development of Mind as the unfolding in Time of an absolute Principle existing eternally for itself. Cf. Hegel's idea of history as the process of a gradual self-recognition of the Objective Mind of the World Spirit.

41 This is an interpretation of what is meant by "neighbor" whom "you shall love as yourself (Leviticus 19:18).

42 The Hebrew Bible uses two principal names for God: YHWH and Elohim. Rabbinic Judaism interprets the former to indicate "the attribute of love," the latter, "the attribute of justice."

43 Deuteronomy 30:14.

44 The following analysis of the holidays touches upon a theme which Rosenzweig elaborated in *The Star of Redemption*. There, the Jewish feasts and the structure of the sacred year are interpreted in the first book of the third part, the Christian feasts and liturgy in the second book of the third part.

45 Friedrich Schiller (1759-1805), the poet, wrote the treatise "Grace and Dignity" and "Letters upon the Aesthetic Education of Man."

46 An allusion to Genesis 1:5: "And there was evening and there was morning, one day."

47 The term "asking" [*Bitte*] should be understood as including petition, prayer, entreaty.

48 Psalm 69:2.

49 Psalm 22:1.

50 Psalm 150:6.

52 This concluding chapter — on death — stands in a striking contrast to the final passage of *The Star of Redemption,* which reads as follows:

"In the innermost sanctuary of divine truth man expects that all the world and his own self will sink down before what he is about to behold. But man beholds only a countenance like to that of his own. The Star of Redemption has become countenance that looks upon me and from which I myself look out. Not God but divine truth has become my mirror.

God, who is the last and the first, has opened for me the portals of the sanctuary that stands in the innermost center. He has allowed himself to be seen. He led me up to that boundary line of life where this vision is vouchsafed. For no man who beholds him may stay within the sphere of life. Hence the sanctuary where he allowed me to behold him had to be a sphere above the world within the world, a life beyond life. But that which he let me see in the beyond of life is nothing more than that which I was already able to perceive in the midst of life itself. Save that now I can see with my eyes what before I could perceive only with my ears.

The vision vouchsafed on the heights of that redeemed sphere above the world opens to me what has already been given by the word of revelation pronounced in the midst of life. To walk in the light of the divine countenance is granted only to him who follows after the words of the divine mouth. Because: 'He hath told thee, O man, what is good, and what the Lord doth require of thee: Only to do justly and to be good at heart and to walk humbly with thy God' [Micah 6:8].

This ultimate word is nothing that is ultimate but something that is eternally near, the nearest to man; it is not the last thing but the first. How difficult is such a first beginning. How difficult is all beginning. To do justly and to be good at heart — that might be as a goal. Before a goal is reached, man's will may desire to pause, and to catch its breath. But 'to walk humbly with thy Lord' — this is no longer a goal, but a thing unconditioned, unconstrained by any conditions, by delay and postponement to a later day; it is a thing wholly related to this very day and so wholly eternal as life itself, and thus as life itself unconditionally a part of the eternal truth.

To walk humbly with thy God: here nothing more is demanded from man than unmediated trust. Trust is, indeed, a great word. It is the seed out of which grow faith, hope and love; and it is the fruit that ripens out of faith, hope and love.

Truth is the simplest of all things and hence the most difficult. It dares, at any moment at all, to acknowledge truth. To walk humbly with thy God: these are the words inscribed over the door through which man leaves the divine sanctuary together with its mysteriously wonderful light, the sanctuary in which no man can remain and live.

But to where does the door open? Do you not know? It opens into Life."

53 Henri Bergson (1859–1941) was opposed to materialist mechanism; he taught that *time* holds the essence of reality. He said: "A true *empiricism is* one that sets itself the task of getting as close as possible to the original" (*Introduction to Metaphysics,* p. 14). Much against Rosenzweig's new thinking, Bergson taught that God is limited by matter and thus finite, and that God and Life are one.

ACKNOWLEDGMENTS

*Heartfelt thanks are due to the officers of The Noonday Press
and especially to Cecil Hemley and Arthur A. Cohen who have
given this book their enthusiasm and ingenious counsel.*

*By his profound knowledge and insight Professor Fritz Kauf-
mann has aided the editor while he was working on the philosophical portions of* Franz Rosenzweig: His Life and Thought; *
his advice graciously given at that time has also been used for
the preparation of this volume.*

The original translation of Understanding the Sick and the
Healthy, *on which the present version is based, was prepared
by T. Luckman.*

*A copy of the author's typescript was provided by the late
Dr. Ernst Baumann of Johannesburg. The photograph of Franz
Rosenzweig's death mask was made by Egone of Boston, Mass.
Much of the typing was done and other assistance affection-
ately rendered by the editor's son Daniel and his daughter Judy.*

December 25, 1886   Born in Cassel, Germany.

1905 to 1912   Study of medicine, later of modern history and philosophy under Jonas Cohn, Friedrich Meinecke and Heinrich Rickert.

1913 to 1914   Quest for religious certainty. Intention of conversion to Christianity. After the experience of an Atonement Day service: decision to remain a Jew. Jewish studies mainly under Hermann Cohen. Discovery of a Schelling philosophical program.

1914 to 1919   War service mainly at the Balkan battle front. Correspondence on the theological issues with Eugen Rosenstock-Huessy. Writing of a Central European educational program; of a treatise on the reconstruction of Jewish learning and education *(It Is Time,* Zeit ist's). Contact with East European Jews (Warsaw). Writing of *The Star of Redemption,* system of religious philosophy.

1920 to 1922   Marriage to Edith Hahn. Foundation of a House of Jewish Studies (Freies Jüdisches Lehrhaus) in Frankfort on the Main. Publication of *Hegel and the State* (Hegel und der Staat). Writing of *Understanding the Sick and the Healthy* (Büchlein vom gesunden und kranken Menschenverstand). Outbreak of a progressive paralysis. Birth of a son, Rafael.

1923 to 1929 Years of paralysis. Ability to speak and to write ceases entirely; stoppage of all movement of limbs. Use of an especially constructed typewriter. Adjustment to life under adverse conditions. Work on translation of Poetry of Judah ha-Levi. Translation of the Bible, with Martin Buber. Essays on religious philosophy, education, biblical and historical problems. Voluminous correspondence.

December 10, 1929 Died in Frankfort.

The definitive editions of Rosenzweig's writings, with the exception of the Hegel book, were published by the Schocken Verlag:

Hegel und der Staat (Hegel and the State). 2 vols. Munich and Berlin 1920.

Der Stern der Erlösung (The Star of Redemption). First edition, Frankfort on the Main 1921. Second edition, Frankfort, 1930.

Die Schrift (Translation of the Bible; together with Martin Buber). 10 volumes (Genesis to Isaiah). Berlin 1925 seq.

Jehuda Halevi (92 poems of Judah ha-Levi; translation and commentary). Berlin 1927.

Briefe (Letters). Edited by Edith Rosenzweig with the cooperation of Ernst Simon. Berlin 1935.

Die Schrift und ihre Verdeutschung (Essays on the Bible translation and interpretation, by Martin Buber and Franz Rosenzweig). Berlin 1936.

Kleinere Schriften (Collected Writings). Berlin 1937.

Franz Rosenzweig: His Life and Thought. Presented by Nahum N. Glatzer. Schocken and Farrar, Straus and Young. New York 1953.